face it

From the Reviewers

"Kyle began teaching me about acne at his parents' home in 2012. The lecture continues in *Face It*. I have no doubt Kyle's efforts to heal himself will help countless thousands of young people to live a more confident, vibrant life. *Face It* provides easy-to-follow, evidence-based acne solutions that can empower even the most discouraged teenagers and adults to take control of their skin health. Let's face it, this manual should be on every high schooler's reading list!"

Adam C. Miller, DDS, MD
Facial Cosmetic Surgeon and Age Management Consult U.S. and Asia
Director, Integrative and Aesthetic Medicine, Malaysia

"Acne medications usually come with terrible side effects. Kyle offers simple, natural remedies and supplements to heal the root cause of your acne and enjoy perfect skin! He has been there and now has great skin, so he understands what you're going through. I trust his advice and love his natural approach for achieving beautiful skin without the use of dangerous medications."

Suzy Cohen, RPh
The Natural Pharmacist, author of *Thyroid Healthy*

"As a physician I've treated many cases of acne in teenagers and young adults in their twenties and know the difficulty in convincing most young people to give up unhealthy 'convenience' foods. Kyle accurately points out that nutrition and supplementation are important parts of the acne puzzle, plus he covers the gambit from history, causes, spot treatments, pharmaceutical treatments, and finally details the scientifically validated approach he used to develop a program to cure his own acne. The conventional medical establishment approaches this problem with antibiotics to kill off the bacteria, which, in turn, further destabilizes the GI tract. As Kyle spells out in his book, there is a better way through nutrition and sound topical solutions. His way, incidentally, will also create good health overall. I encourage teens, those in their twenties, or adults suffering with acne to follow the advice he's written in his book."

Dr. Patrick Purdue, D.O.M.

"Trapped in the conundrum of acne is unfortunately a commonplace for many people, especially teens. Kyle Craichy has demonstrated that there is HOPE with this meticulously researched book. More importantly, through his candid humility by revealing his own story and experience, he provides a solution with strategies based on scientific evidence. I applaud Kyle for searching and exposing truths and myths about acne that can help so many. His inclusion of the social and emotional struggles an individual goes through with severe acne shows a heart of mercy and compassion for others. I have prayed for extraordinary blessings to cover and carry this book!"

Tamara Mariea, PhD, CCN

"Kyle Craichy shares his personal travails with severe acne and along the way discovers that the medical experts helping him were doing more harm than good. Rather than giving up in defeat, he takes inspiration from his father, KC Craichy, and dives headlong into research to discover the true causes and the real remedies that too few know about! *Face It* is an extraordinarily well-researched book that reveals what few dermatologists will tell you about acne's origin. You will be profoundly satisfied with the comprehensive view from both beneath the skin and above it, along with the many nutritional options not taught in medical schools. Put what Kyle uncovers in *Face It* to the test and you, too, can find yourself free from acne!"

Robert Scott Bell, D.A. Hom.
Coauthor of *Unlock the Power to Heal*

"I just finished reading *Face It*, which brought back some less than pleasant memories from my own teenage years, and I was very impressed by Kyle's ability to speak to his own challenges and how he overcame them through his fascinating research. The book is an easy and interesting read. But more importantly, the information that Kyle presents is founded in science, which makes his recommendations even more powerful. I highly recommend this book for anyone who has had challenges with acne and for anyone who is interested in having healthier skin."

Greg Wells, PhD
Author of *Superbodies: Peak Performance Secrets from the World's Best Athletes*

"Kyle Craichy is an amazing young man. I met him twelve years ago when he became one of my martial arts students. He excelled in his studies and earned his 2nd Degree Black Belt after seven years of intense focus, self-discipline, and hard work. Those are the same qualities that make him a great entrepreneur and wonderful friend. Kyle grew up in a loving family that has helped him and his brothers and sisters love others even as Christ loves them. He learned from his parents the importance of superfood nutrition and natural health, which helped Kyle find the answers to his personal questions about skin care. *Face It* is about HOPE. God gives us hope in every aspect of our life and that includes the health of our skin. I know the information in this book will make a big difference in your life and the lives of everyone who reads it."

Mark McGee
Yon Ch'uan Martial Arts

"There is hardly anything more traumatic to anyone's self-confidence than to struggle with the physical and emotional scars caused by acne. Yet almost everyone fights this battle! So why is there no effective approach to healthy skin readily available? Answer: There is! Kyle Craichy presents the results of his own groundbreaking research and the answers he discovered that took him all the way from victim to victor in the war on acne. I recommend this to anyone who suffers from acne."

John Peterson, ND
Founder of Living Strength Transformation Systems

face it

Winning the War on Acne

Like · Comment · Share

LIVINGFUEL
PUBLISHING
TAMPA, FLORIDA

kyle craichy

Face It: Winning the War on Acne

Copyright © 2014 by Kyle Craichy

ISBN 978-0-9763602-1-6

Published by Living Fuel Publishing. You can reach us on the Internet at www.livingfuel.com or call 1-866-580-FUEL.

Literary development and cover/interior design by Koechel Peterson & Associates, Inc., Minneapolis, Minnesota.

Manufactured in the United States of America

I DEDICATE THIS BOOK

to my Lord and Savior Jesus Christ.

My people perish for lack of knowledge.
Hosea 4:6

Thank You for the knowledge
You have helped me acquire.
For Your Glory

acknowledgments

Papa, I want to thank you for absolutely everything you have done for me. You are my greatest inspiration, and I am so grateful for everything you have taught and helped me with.

Mom, thank you for always being willing to take the time out of your busy days to help me with everything I am working on and for always being there for me.

Austin and Sarah, thank you for being my chief test subjects and always giving me your honest feedback. Your thoughts have helped me greatly and all the input in smells, textures, looks—everything.

Grace and Joshua, you guys are amazing, and your knowledge is so advanced beyond your years. Thank you for always being willing to give your opinions and for all the love and support you have given me, pushing me to be better.

Leonard Smith MD, you are awesome and an amazing resource. Thank you for the wealth of knowledge you have imparted to me and for taking your valuable time to help make this book the best it can possibly be.

Ty Bollinger, you are a big inspiration to me—you research the truth and tell as many people as you possibly can about it to help set them free. To have you backing me means a lot. Thank you.

Dr. Robert Scott Bell, Dr. Suzy Cohen, Dr. Patrick Purdue, Dr. Tamara Mariea, and Dr. Greg Wells, I want to thank each of you for your time, encouragement, and support. It is very encouraging and motivating to have people of your statuses believe in me as you do.

Finally, I want to thank all the people who let me test my formulations on them. You all played a huge part in helping a lot of people clear their skin as we have. PTL for you guys. Your trust in me and in the things I came up with motivates me.

contents

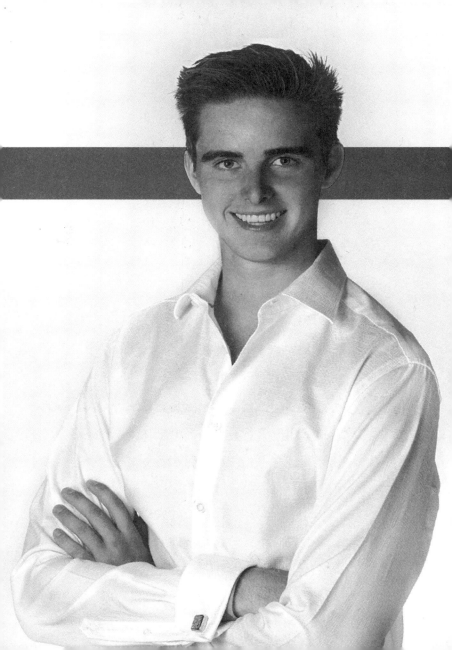

about kyle craichy

As a health researcher and educator with a focus on skin health, Kyle Craichy is Founder and CEO of LXR Organics, Inc., an organic personal care company. He is a lead singer/musician in the Orchestral R&B group, KAJ Brothers. Kyle is accomplished beyond his years, having grown up in his parents' superfood nutrition company, Living Fuel. After completing his accelerated entrepreneurial internship at Living Fuel with the same diligence that he used to become an award-winning classical pianist, a second-degree black belt in martial arts, and as quarterback leading his football team to the state championship game, he commenced his intensive acne research project to solve his own acne challenges.

foreword

I t is my pleasure and honor to endorse Kyle's book, *Face It*. He has done a masterful job of creating a book that includes the history, personal testimony, psychological issues, diet, nutritional science, and practical solutions to know and use when dealing with acne. I was so impressed with Kyle's work that it seemed as though it was written by a doctor who had completed a comprehensive functional medicine course on the subject of acne.

Speaking from his personal experience and an impressive array of research, Kyle takes the reader through his journey of finding a way of successfully combating his struggles with acne. Challenging the "myths" of conventional treatments with their risky side effects, he strikes out into a search of unconventional healthy options that have led him down an enlightened path to skin wellness. He empathically shares with others in an informal yet informed way that can be enjoyed by teenagers and adults alike.

The book was so engaging for me that I was stimulated to read even more in terms of the science of acne, and it is fascinating. As Kyle clearly points out, acne is multifactorial, and what you see on the skin is only a reflection of much deeper issues in the tissues. These issues include blood sugar, hormones, mineral deficiencies, and much more. The book helps to bring forward the twenty-first-century approach to health, which is a functional, systematic approach that leads to a cure rather than merely controlling the symptoms. Anyone who chooses to follow the recommendations of *Face It* will likely not only rid themselves of the curse of acne but also enjoy a much healthier and happy life.

Dr. Leonard Smith, MD
Author and Integrative Medicine Expert

I have come that they may have life,
and that they may have it more abundantly.

Jesus Christ, John 10:10

preface

This book achieves a breakthrough for anyone seeking the root causes and lifelong solutions for acne. Beyond the chemical poisons pushed by product manufacturers, there's a far more natural and healthy way to discover healthy, clean skin. Kyle Craichy's book is a voice of wisdom and reason in a world that's full of poison and toxicity.

Mike Adams
The Health Ranger, editor of NaturalNews.com

introduction

Do you remember pimples? You know . . . acne? I certainly do. Nothing was more embarrassing than to wake up, get ready for school, look in the mirror, and realize that I had an outbreak on my face or back. I'm forty-six years old as I write this, but I still remember those days.

Face It will take you on an expedition with a brilliant twenty-year-old young man, Kyle Craichy, who took the bull by the horns and decided to find out why, despite eating an organic diet and living an active and healthy lifestyle, he still had horrible outbreaks of acne. Craichy begins the journey in ancient Egypt, takes the reader to Greece, then Rome, then culminates in the modern era as he documents the history of acne treatments and explains why none of them really worked very well.

In this book, the author explains exactly what acne is (something most people still don't understand), the different types of acne, the process of inflammation, and succinctly elucidates the multiple factors (hormonal, environmental, and hygienic) that impact this dreadful skin disorder, while addressing the emotional and physical scarring that oftentimes results from the "acne wars."

Craichy does a masterful job of illuminating the reader about essential nutrition, essential oils, and proper supplementation. But Craichy doesn't leave you hanging! In the end, he provides the reader with a step-by-step road map on how to use hydration, proper sleep, nutrition, exercise, supplementation, and essential oils to say goodbye to acne once and for all.

As a health researcher, I was quite impressed with the voluminous amounts of research that Craichy performed in order to write this remarkable book—quite a feat for a young man whose counterparts are stereotypically "partying" in college. This book is an important book for everyone's library. I highly recommend that you obtain your copy today. You won't be sorry.

Ty M. Bollinger
Author and Researcher

The doctor of the future will give no medicine, but will interest his patients in the care of the human frame, in diet, and in the cause and prevention of disease.

Thomas Alva Edison

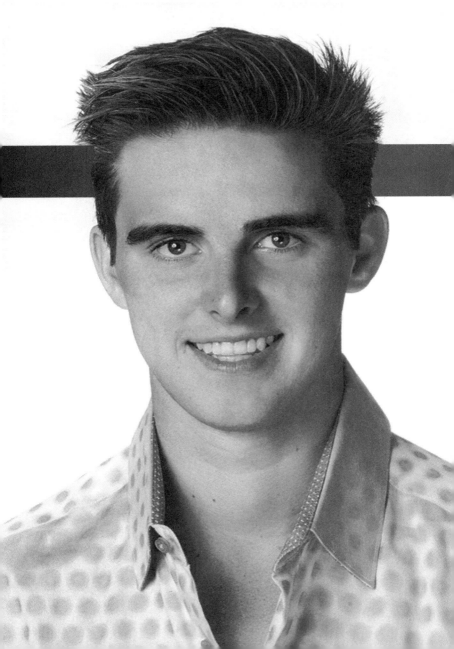

chapter 1

My Story

Dear friend, let me tell you a story . . . my story.

A short time ago, I felt anxious beyond anything I had ever experienced before. Why? Because I was almost nineteen and still struggling with an acne problem. In fact, it only appeared to be getting worse. We're not talking about just any ol' acne . . . no, this was severe acne. The type of cringe-worthy acne that appears on the computer screen when you type "acne" into Google Images and then thank God that it isn't you being shown in the photos you find.

It was the acne of my nightmares that I never thought would actually happen to me. But it did! And it was one of the worst and most challenging problems that I ever had to deal with. The problem was—no acne treatment I tried ever really worked, at least not long term.

Granted, before I developed severe acne, I had dealt with mild to moderate acne breakouts since I was about sixteen. And like most people who've experienced acne, I spent hundreds and hundreds of dollars on all sorts of creams, lotions, and prescription medications that in the end essentially amounted to nothing more than a waste of money.

Every time I tried something new, my hopes would soar, thinking that finally this was the breakthrough product that would be the end of my troubles. The truth is, some products worked for brief periods of time, but the acne always came back. Some treatments, however, made the acne worse. I got to the point where I just couldn't handle the disappointment anymore. Like tens of thousands of other people, I felt as though I had tried everything and was running out of options. In one continuous, unrelenting swipe, it tore at my self-esteem, self-worth, happiness, and quality of life.

> *I got to the point where I just couldn't handle the disappointment anymore.*

Let me give you an example of what I'm referring to and see if you can relate.

Just over three years ago (I was seventeen), a birthday party was held for one of my friends at his folks' beach place in St. Petersburg, Florida. When I got there, everyone was already down chilling on the beach, throwing the football, playing volleyball, etc. Still in my street clothes, I joined in the fun. After a while, we decided it would be fun to get into the pool, so I jumped in, clothes and all, under the excuse of "not wanting to go upstairs to change into my swimsuit." Truthfully, that had nothing to do with it. In fact, I was too embarrassed, humiliated, and ashamed of a fresh terrible outbreak of "bacne" to take my shirt off in front of my friends. Because they all knew that I worked out and had an athletic, muscular body, they wondered, *What's the deal with Kyle?*

The truth is I was more than just a little frustrated. I was exasperated! I wanted straight answers on acne, and I wasn't getting any. Not only that, but much of the information I received proved to be untrue. For example, some of today's dermatologists tell kids that diet and nutrition have "little or nothing to do with breakouts." I read that time after time, from one source after another, and it's absolutely false. The real question should be, *Is nutrition the only thing or even the most important thing?* And just as important, *Is there anything else you need to do besides just learning to eat right?* I deal with these questions and many others that are directly related in this book.

Here is a point that needs to be made as it relates to nutrition. There is no doubt that superior nutrition will help accelerate healing after breakouts and will even go a long way to help prevent them from occurring in the first place. Likewise, bad nutrition can trigger outbreaks or make them much worse. Nevertheless, there are other important factors to take into consideration if you want to prevent future outbreaks and ultimately eliminate acne from your life.

As important as nutrition is, it is not the only thing. I know that from firsthand experience. In my case, I have always had the best nutrition on the planet. My parents' company is Living Fuel, the leader in Superfood Nutrition, so for my whole life I have had the best natural nutrition one could have. Believe it or not, I've never had a donut or eaten at McDonald's my entire life. I don't eat fried foods, don't drink soda or alcohol, and sugar (only natural sugar) has been at a minimum. Plus, I grew up giving my body the nutrients, vitamins, minerals, and other macro and micronutrients it needs through Living Fuel. But I STILL HAD ACNE!

So obviously, there has to be something in addition to nutrition; but what is it?

The Desperate Repeating Cycle

In this book, I explore all the other possible causes so you can personally discover the main causes for your own breakouts. In my case, for instance, I discovered that I would breakout worse when I was working out really hard. This is due to spikes in testosterone and other male hormones that are activated as part of muscle metabolism. And, yes, I have heard the same from numerous athletes.

This brings up an important point. Due to my dad's influence (he is 6'4" and 220 pounds of muscle), I have worked out all my life, but when I was sixteen, I got really serious and stepped it up. I started lifting heavy and running sprints. I played football and basketball, so I trained hard. It became obvious that the harder I worked out and the more I pushed myself, the more I broke out, especially on my back and shoulders. I made that connection, but like thousands of others, I didn't know what to do, so I dealt with it as so many others do and bounced from one acne product to another acne product. None of them worked for me, and my problem worsened. In fact, my back was as badly broken out as I've seen on anyone, and my facial breakouts would come and go every so often. It was frustrating socially and a huge embarrassment!

No one wants to be seen with "flawed" skin. And even though a lot of my teammates and friends had acne as well, I doubt that anyone sees other people's acne as bad as their own, so I struggled with every breakout, felt alone, and couldn't stand to be seen without a shirt on even though I was in good shape. It got so bad that whenever I was in the locker room with my teammates, instead of changing at my locker like everyone else, I would go to the bathroom and change in one of the stalls.

> *I struggled with every breakout, felt alone, and couldn't stand to be seen without a shirt on even though I was in good shape.*

The point of sharing all this is that having acne affects what we do, and it affects our self-image and self-confidence. For me it was a constant reminder to keep a shirt on and have my hair in my face to cover my acne-ridden forehead. Perhaps we shouldn't care that much, but we do, and despite parents and dermatologists telling us not to pop the pimples because it will make it worse, we do because there is no way we are going out in public with a bunch of pimples on our face or back. It's the weirdest feeling, but when you see or feel you have a pimple, your body wants to pop it so badly that it is impossible not to. For some reason we see our own pimples bigger and brighter than they really are. Even though others might not even notice a lone pimple on our chin, we feel like it is a bright flashing neon sign attracting attention. So I did what everyone else does—

pop them, which spreads the bacteria, makes the breakout worse, and bruises and scars the heck out of my skin. The cycle kept repeating, causing an out-of-control situation, and since none of the major products were working for me and just drying my skin out, there was little hope for me other than waiting it out.

When I became eighteen years old, the acne was still bad and growing worse for all the extra testosterone going through my body as a result of growth spurts and working out harder. I graduated from high school and the problem remained as bad as ever. I felt as though I had tried every remedy, and everything out there had the same concept! DRY OUT THE OILS! Bouncing from one product to the next, each product made my skin drier and yet the pimples did not go away. After doing this method for close to two and a half years, my face and back were so dry that they looked unhealthy. *I had had enough.*

The Turning Point

Meanwhile, I had always been afraid of using oils on my skin for fear of breaking out worse. But one night as I was getting ready for bed, I decided to try a shea butter lotion/cream (a complex fat extracted from the nut of the African shea tree) that was in my bathroom drawer. I was hesitant at first, because it went

> *I knew right then that the conventional methods I had tried had flaws and much of the philosophies about what caused acne and what helped it simply weren't true.*

against everything I had been taught about treating acne, but I ended up applying it, and the next morning my skin looked healthier than it had in a long time. Not only that, but there was a reduction in the swelling of the zits. I knew right then that the conventional methods I had tried had flaws and much of the philosophies about what caused acne and what helped it simply weren't true. They were actually myths.

So I kept lathering the cream on my back and face each morning and evening, and after several days I started to have some minor breakouts. I found I was using too much of it and putting it on too thick to where my skin was constantly greasy and not able to absorb it all, so it just sat there on my skin clogging pores. I realized that there is a limit and too much of a good thing is a bad thing. I reduced the amount I applied and had some dramatic results in the overall healthiness of my skin and also had a slight reduction in acne.

That was really the turning point for me in researching acne treatment in unconventional ways. I discovered that the application of moisture and oils to the skin is not harmful, but they are helpful to keeping your skin looking moist and plump.

The Search Begins

That began my search for what oils are the best. And I told my dad I wanted to come up with something to fix my acne, so he gave me stacks and stacks of research books and articles that he had accumulated during his years as a health and nutrition researcher. I devoured them and found many others, making notes of my own and going through the different information. Through trial and error, mixing different natural ingredients together, I tried the things that seemed compelling, slowly finding what worked and what didn't work for me. I would try anything I found research on (except the drugs, because all the studies showed dangerous consequences) to get rid of this age-old problem. I researched the history of acne, what acne actually really is, the causes of acne, methods to treat it, drugs versus natural methods, acne myths—anything I could find.

That is what birthed this book. I compiled the research and cut out anything that didn't work to discover the system that healed my back and face and made my skin beautiful again. It is amazing how the skin works, and that most of the same nutrients that work for one issue tend to be effective to treat another issue. While my focus was on acne, my discoveries actually result in youthful skin for people who don't have acne. My mother has become the biggest fan of this discovery, and she says that variations of my acne formulas are the "best thing" she's ever used on her skin. She is so excited about them that she strongly requests that my next project be focused on anti-aging skin and skin health for her and countless others who don't have acne, so stay tuned. . . .

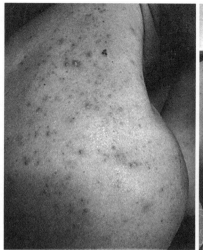 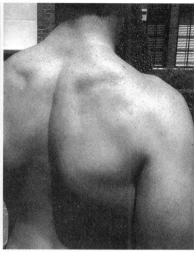

before

after
(10 weeks later)

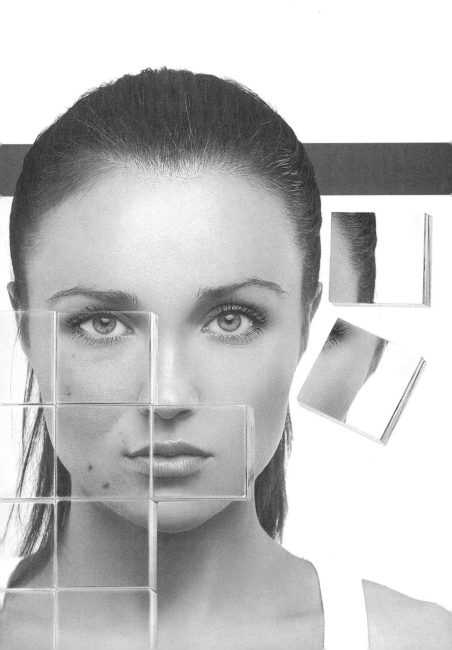

chapter 2
A Short History of Acne

If you think, as many do today, that acne is a recent historical development brought on by poor diets, pollution, or lack of exercise, think again. Acne has been written about since ancient times, including prescriptions for its treatment.

For instance, ancient Egyptian writings mention that several pharaohs suffered with acne. Not surprisingly, given their culture, superstitions were given for the cause of breakouts, such as telling lies, and magic, spells, and charms were offered as treatments. If your experience with acne has been anything like mine, you might feel desperate enough to try magic or a charm or two. In the Ebers Papyrus (dating to c. 1550 B.C.), the word *aku-t* is cited that was later translated as "boils, blains, sores, pustules, or any inflammatory swelling," and some of its remedies are mentioned as animal origin preparations and honey.[1]

In ancient Greece, the earliest description of acne appeared in the writings of the Byzantine physician Aetius Amidenus (mid-fifth century to mid-sixth century).[2] The word *acne* appears to have evolved from the Greek word *acme*, which means "point or spot."[3] From the historical records, both Hippocrates (c. 460–370 B.C.) and Aristotle (c. 384–322 B.C.) were aware of this illness. Aristotle wrote about this condition in detail.[4] The ancient Greeks knew acne as *tovoot*. According to the meaning of this word in the singular as "the first growth of the beard," it was associated with puberty. Around A.D. 2, the meaning of acne appeared to be widened to include the highest point of growth and development, and thus puberty. It was recommended that honey be used for softer lesions and a mixture in soap base for harder ones.[5]

In ancient Rome, acne was often treated with baths, using hot mineral water combined with sulfur to unclog and cleanse pores as well as dry out oils that clogged the skin. A. Cornelius Celsius (c. 25 B.C.–A.D. 50), a Roman encyclopaedist, mentioned this treatment in his medical book titled *De Medicina*: "To treat pimples and spots and freckles is almost a waste of time, yet women cannot be torn away from caring for their looks. But of these just mentioned, pimples and spots are commonly known, although that species of spot is rare which is called by the Greeks *semion*, since it is rather red and irregular. But pimples are best removed by the application of resin to

> *In ancient Rome, acne was often treated with baths, using hot mineral water combined with sulfur to unclog and cleanse pores as well as dry out oils that clogged the skin.*

which not less than the same amount of split alum and a little honey has been added."[6]

Until the 1800s, people did not discover any more useful treatments against acne and have continuously used sulfur because they saw it can dry and exfoliate the skin.

Dr. William H. Schuessler, a nineteenth-century German medical doctor, did studies that led to a list of 12 biochemic cell salts. He concluded that any deficiencies in the body's cell salts resulted in illness, including acne. He believed it was necessary to restore the correct balance of tissue salts for removing acne blemishes. His cell salt therapies, first discovered in 1873, are still practiced by some homeopaths around the world.

In 1902, doctors used X-rays as a form of acne treatment. This may seem crazy to you, but even today a similar treatment called blue light therapy is used.

In 1920, Jack Breitbart of the Revlon Corporation first developed benzoyl peroxide, which is still used today in the treatment to kill acne bacteria.[7] It works as a peeling agent, increasing skin turnover, clearing pores, and reducing the bacterial count. It is typically applied to the affected areas in gel or cream form, in concentrations of 2.5 percent and increasing through 5 percent and up to 10 percent.

In 1930, laxatives were used for treating the condition called "chastity pustules." Some people thought that virgins could not eliminate toxins from their bodies because they did not have any sexual contact, so they tried using laxatives against acne. Today's

> *In 1930, laxatives were used for treating the condition called "chastity pustules."*

doctors know that having sex has nothing to do with eliminating toxins, but they recognize that constipation can be a cause of acne as toxins accumulate in the body.

In 1950, antibiotics were used in treating acne caused by germs. Tetracycline, for instance, was used with great results, but nowadays it is no longer used as it has lost its effect against some skin germs. Other more powerful antibiotics have taken its place.

In 1960, Tretinoin (the carboxylic acid form of vitamin A), also known as Retin A, was discovered to have a beneficial effect against acne. Later on, the oral isotretionine was made and the battle against acne became easier. These products are still used nowadays with the same effects on acne.

Keep in mind that I am only presenting this as a history of attempts to deal with acne. I am not condoning any of them, as all of them have differing degrees of negative side effects that I could never recommend as worth whatever benefit they might bring, especially the next one.

In the 1980s, Accutane (a member of a family of compounds known as retinoids that are related to vitamin A) appeared in the American market. It was considered a breakthrough treatment on serious acne but came with a host of side effects worse than the acne itself and was taken off the market in 2009. Today, its generic knockoff isotretinoin products can have extremely serious side effects—mental health problems, including depression, psychosis, and suicide, and when taken by pregnant women, miscarriage or birth defects—that I'll deal more extensively with in Chapter Eight.

In 1990, laser therapy made its first steps in treating acne. Lasers work on the premise of exciting compounds called porphyrins, which live inside acne bacteria. When the lasers excite the porphyrins, the porphyrins damage the bacteria wall, effectively killing the bacteria, which should reduce the symptoms of the acne. The process is quite expensive, and researchers suggest that its effectiveness is short-term.[8]

Blue light therapy was developed for treating acne in the 2000's followed by studies that were done by different medical groups in the United States and Europe. Treatment for acne using blue light therapy involves using a narrow high-intensity light. Machines can be used at home to help acne patients obtain a clear complexion, although its effectiveness shows mixed results similar to laser therapy. Neither are cures.

Microneedling with dermaroller has emerged as a novel treatment of acne scars. Orentreich first described subcision or dermal needling in 1995 for scars, and in 2006, Fernandes developed percutaneous collagen induction therapy with the dermaroller.[9]

So how much improvement have they made on this issue over the years? We find that each generation seemingly got closer, but have they really? It doesn't matter if I walk down the streets of Orlando, New York, Paris, London, or Rome, acne is everywhere, and the problem seems to be worse than ever, and it's not limited to teenagers. The evolution of acne treatments has also added potentially deadly side effects that show how bad the issue really is—that people are willing to risk their health and even their lives in order to be rid of it by doing some of these treatments.

So did any of them have it right? Do we have it right today? In looking for new ways, have we looked in the wrong places for solutions? We have been looking for ways to treat the symptoms with drugs and drying without looking at treating the issues that cause acne in the first place.

> *In looking for new ways, have we looked in the wrong places for solutions?*

But I discipline my body and
bring it into subjection ...

The Apostle Paul, 1 Corinthians 9:27

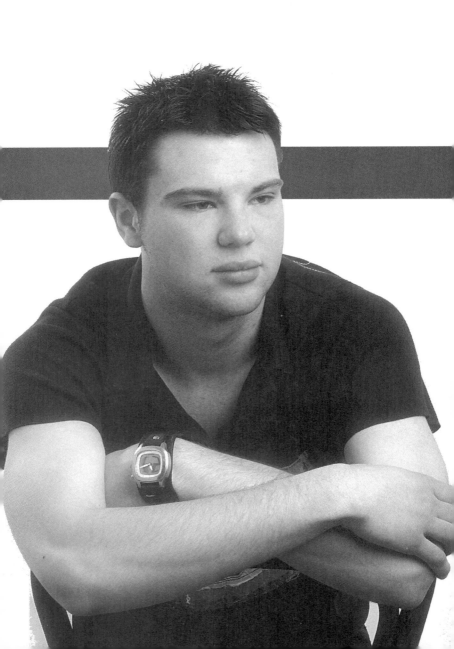

chapter 3
You Are Not Alone

While you may feel just as incredibly alone as I did, acne is the most widespread skin disease in the world, with millions and millions of sufferers. The adolescent years are the most common and notorious for acne breakouts, affecting 80 to 90 percent of teenagers to some degree, even supermodels.[10] We hope that any breakout is mild and short-lived, but they can be severe and disfiguring. If you are among the fortunate ones, acne's prevalence declines over time and tends to disappear or at least decrease by age 25.[11] There is, however, no way to know when or if it will disappear or if it will disappear entirely, and it's pos-

> *The adolescent years are the most common and notorious for acne breakouts, affecting 80 to 90 percent of teenagers to some degree.*

sible that you are among the unfortunate individuals who contend with this condition well into their thirties, forties, and beyond.[12] It's not what any of us want to be told, I know, and it's one of the reasons I decided I had to seek a therapy that would work for me.

Adult acne is a far more universal problem than you might think. Among adult women, about 50 percent experience acne breakouts at some point; among men, about 25 percent[13]—and the chronic nature of the condition means adults may endure symptoms for decades. As is true of adolescent acne, adult acne is often caused by a hormonal imbalance. Many women, for instance, break out every month at the onset of their period, and acne is a common symptom of PMS.

Acne is also associated with polycystic ovarian syndrome (PCOS), a hormonal condition that causes irregular or absent menstrual periods due to ovulation irregularities. In women over 35, the hormonal fluctuations that orchestrate their periods tend to become more dramatic and unpredictable as they enter perimenopause and approach menopause, which can aggravate hormonal acne. Many women who haven't had a breakout since their teens or early twenties suddenly find themselves battling acne in their forties.

And if you think those who are considered the elite in beauty somehow escape the acne wars, just listen to supermodels and Hollywood stars and celebrities. They may always look fabulous on the screen, but that is thanks to makeup artists and airbrushing. The main difference between their battle and yours is that they cannot let their breakouts and imperfections be seen. To cover up the problem, some of them find a foundation that is appropriate to their skin color and has a high pigment concentration while others use two layers of foundation separated by a layer of transparent face powder.

From supermodels such as Cindy Crawford to singers Celine Dion, Ricky Martin, Britney Spears, and Seal to actresses Julia Stiles, Thandie Newton, and Winona Ryder to actors Richard Burton and Kevin Bacon, the battle goes on. Here are a few comments from the stars themselves:

- "When I was in high school and I had acne, I spent a lot of time sulking in my room. I was depressed. I was not happy."—*Adam Levine*[14]

- "I had bad hormonal acne when I was 17 . . . then, I had stress acne when I was 20, which they kindly video-airbrushed out of the movie. But I realized how debilitating and embarrassing it can be to have cystic acne."—*Emma Stone told Refinery29.com*[15]

- "I used to have very bad acne, so bad I wanted to commit suicide over it."—*Ethan Hawke*[16]

- "I'm incredibly self-conscious about the fact that I get bad skin."—*Keira Knightley told Australian Vogue*[17]

- "I had acne as a teen, and it made me so insecure to be on camera—not a good thing when you are on a television series."—*Kaley Cuoco*[18]

- "I have acne scars. I'm self-conscious about that, so sometimes I wear too much makeup to cover them up."—*Katy Perry told Cosmopolitan*[19]

- "I have the same breakouts as everybody else." —*Scarlett Johansson told Elle*[20]

- "I'm basically a sexless geek. Look at me, I have pasty white skin, I have acne scars, and I'm five-foot-nothing."—*Mike Myers*[21]

- "I always have to carry concealer in my makeup case because I have adult acne."—*Madonna*[22]

- "I've always had a serious pimple problem. It's one of life's trials, right?"—*Cameron Diaz*[23]

- "I hate [pimples] and, of course, I still get them like everyone else."—*Sarah Michelle Gellar*[24]

Even celebrities, who could pay for any treatment, no matter the cost, don't have a solution for this epidemic. Something is wrong with this picture.

Much More to It Than Scarring

If you're a veteran of the acne wars, you know that acne results in the inflammation within the dermis, which leads the body to try to heal the wound. But often too much collagen will end up at that specific breakout site, resulting in scarring.[25] When phrases such as ice pick scars, boxcar scars, rolling scars, or pigmented scars are part of your conversation, you have probably searched and searched for ways to treat the scarring, whether with lasers or microneedling or pure vitamin E oils or other gels or almost anything anyone suggests (the list is very long).

Aside from scarring, though, acne often has a profound effect on one's entire life in a multitude of ways, which may not be understood or appreciated by your family and friends. Acne is particularly troubling because of its visibility and its intimate relationship with our self-esteem. Dr. Steven R. Feldman, professor of dermatology in the Wake Forest University School of Medicine, says, "The skin in general, and particularly the skin of the face, is the way we see ourselves. It's the way others see us, and most importantly, it's the way we *think* others see us."[26] That is the heart of the issue.

In that acne usually is most pronounced during adolescence, when we already tend to be our most insecure, its main effects are psychological, leading to reduced self-esteem, self-confidence, and overall outlook in general.[27] A 2006 study showed that "the more prominent symptoms were embarrassment, impaired self-image, low self-esteem, self-consciousness, frustration, and anger. Some subjects thought that acne had affected their personalities permanently and adversely. Psychological sequelae were attributed to the effects of facial acne on appearance."[28] And as you can imagine or perhaps already know, the emotional scars can remain long after the acne has disappeared.

Even mild breakouts can negatively impact how one feels about himself. That is no surprise, given the many corollary problems it introduces, such as depression, anxiety, personality problems, emotions, self-concept, social isolation, social assertiveness, social anxiety, and body dissatisfaction.[29] What may be surprising to you, though, is that adults are more likely than their adolescent counterparts to feel that acne negatively effects their lives—regardless of how severe their acne is.[30] This may be because their acne has been longer lasting or resistant to treatment or because there is a greater social stigma for adults with acne.

> *Even mild breakouts can negatively impact how one feels about himself.*

Many studies have been done that show that depression and anxiety are more common in those with acne than the general population. Studies have shown that acne patients report deficits in the quality of their lives (the degree of enjoyment or satisfaction experienced in everyday life) as great as those reported by patients with chronic health problems, such as asthma, epilepsy, diabetes, and arthritis.[31] Of particular concern is the rate that acne sufferers of all ages go on to develop anxiety disorders, depression, and other mental disorders, even suicide.[32] Clearly, no one should take the emotional consequences of acne lightly.

When It Leads to Social Withdrawal

In a society that places a phenomenal emphasis on appearance, acne sufferers often feel uncomfortable or embarrassed or even ashamed of their condition. Dr. Jerry Tan, director of the Acne Research and Treatment Centre in Windsor, Canada, says, "While the physical features of acne are readily apparent to us all, the emotional and social impact of acne is often underestimated by non-sufferers. This can be manifested as anxiety, depression, and social withdrawal. . . . Studies have shown that those with acne are dissatisfied with their appearance, embarrassed, self-conscious, and lack self-confidence. Problems with social interactions with the opposite gender, appearances in public, and with strangers have also been observed."[33]

In teenagers, depression may manifest as social withdrawal (the avoidance of peers or the retreat to the bedroom) and/or impaired school performance (lower grades or missed assignments). Something as simple as having a photograph taken with friends or family can become a major issue. It is so easy to get worried that everyone is staring at your pimples that you don't want to leave your house. No matter what reason another person is looking at us, we automatically assume it is because of our acne.

> *Something as simple as having a photograph taken with friends or family can become a major issue.*

However, if we avoid going out, mingling with other people, or being seen in public, we lose out in the things that will help us grow and mature as a person. We lose out on possible social connections, missing out on the opportunities to make friends and learn from other people.

Many people do not participate in exercise or sports because of their acne. For instance, who could blame a young man who avoids swimming due to the blemishes on his chest or back. Dr. Martyn Standage, a lecturer in Great Britain's School for Health at the University of Bath, says, "The skin is the most visible organ in the human body and, as such, is an important part of personal image. Fear of having one's skin evaluated by others has implications for physical and social well-being. Sport and exercise activities provide many opportunities for the skin to be exposed to evaluation. Due to this, acne sufferers may become so anxious about their appearance that it prevents them from participating in physical activity."[34]

A 2006 study conducted at Wake Forest University School of Medicine on social sensitivity and acne determined that "greater acne severity was significantly associated with poorer social outcomes and quality of life. For women, higher social sensitivity was independently associated with poorer outcomes, while for men, higher social sensitivity interacted with acne severity and was associated with worse social outcomes and life quality." Dermatologist Jennifer Krejci-Manwaring concluded that "men and women with severe acne have the most trouble in social interactions with both friends and strangers. However, women who are more sensitive even when their skin is clear have much more difficulty when they have outbreaks."[35]

Some Even Feel a Sense of Guilt and Shame

Adding to this sensitivity, the prevalence of myths regarding acne development may even lead some to feel a sense of guilt or shame, as if they are somehow responsible for their acne. According to the *Dermatology Online Journal*, a study of acne sufferers in dermatological care showed that 30 percent of these patients believed that poor skin hygiene contributed to their acne.[36] The truth is that acne is primarily caused by hormonal changes during puberty, menstruation, pregnancy, and menopause. Unfortunately, believing this hygiene myth causes young people to blame themselves for not keeping their skin perfectly clean, giving them feelings of guilt and shame and stress. The stress of acne makes breakouts even worse, as it has been demonstrated that stress can cause excess oil production.[37] This oil mixes with dead skin cells and skin bacteria resulting in clogged pores and breakouts. It is a vicious cycle, and it keeps getting worse and worse.

Some people end up feeling ugly and undesirable and never pleased with the way they look. They may be smart and intelligent and well liked, but they become oblivious to their assets as though these are meaningless. After a while, a person with acne can become blind to his strengths and focused on his weaknesses. This is detrimental in the long run for they may let opportunities pass them by because of their obsession with their physical appearance.

Unfortunately, it can lead to long-lasting emotional and psychological effects. A person who has intermittent breakouts will often become angrier with every acne eruption. He can also become more obsessed about his condition; his self-esteem can also become lower with every breakout. In the end, even when the acne is all gone and a previously afflicted person's skin has become smooth and clear of acne breakouts, the feelings of inadequacy and undesirability often linger.

It is clear that while acne may be considered "medically simple," it can still be a very harmful condition. It needs to be treated and treated promptly, too, if the negative emotional and psychological effects are to be avoided.

...I will remember that there is art to medicine as well as science, and that warmth, sympathy, and understanding may outweigh the surgeon's knife or the chemist's drug.... I will prevent disease whenever I can, for prevention is preferable to cure.

From the Hippocratic Oath (Modern Version) by Louis Lasagna, Academic Dean of the School of Medicine at Tufts University, written in 1964 and used in many medical schools today.

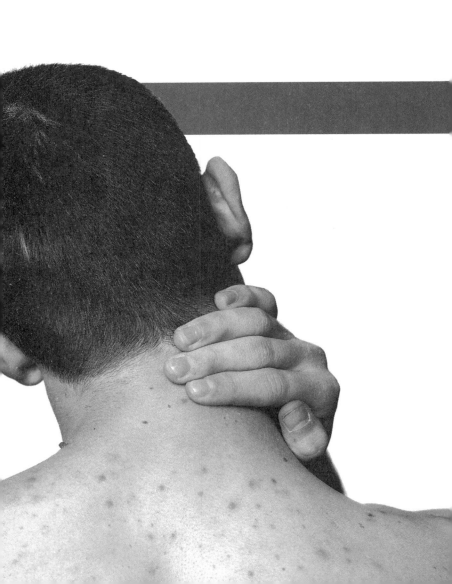

chapter 4

The Amazing Human Body and Acne

In my father's best-selling book, *Super Health*, he stated, "With all its amazing complexities, the human body is easily the most amazing creation in the entire known universe. When King David asserted, 'I will praise You, for I am fearfully and wonderfully made' (Psalm 139:14), he was marveling over all the intricacies of the human body and soul, including the many remarkable immunity and healing systems that we have been lovingly given by our Maker. While our body was designed by God to keep itself in health, the fact is that we are responsible for faithfully supplying it with all it absolutely requires for health. Twenty-four hours a day the trillions of cells in our body must be receiving the right nutrition to function at an optimal level. If we deprive our body of what it requires, or if we abuse our body with what we know or don't know is harmful, we will suffer a breakdown in our health."[38]

The human body is so awesome that it is designed to heal itself. When you scrape your knee, your body starts healing on its own immediately. You can speed up the healing by taking certain vitamins or applying them directly, such as vitamin A or aloe vera gel. The same holds true for your skin, which is the largest organ of your body, and any other part of your body. Your body wants to heal itself, but certain deficiencies of required nutrients can hinder it from doing so. In giving your body these nutrients, you aid your body's healing process. On top of that, if you combine nutrients together, as opposed to taking them alone, these vitamins, minerals, and antioxidants combine like a symphony of healing for the skin. Since all these are a necessity for your skin as well as the rest of your body, they can seem to work together miraculously.

> *The human body is so awesome that it is designed to heal itself.*

It would be marvelous if our bodies worked perfectly to produce perfect skin, but intruders such as acne often break through our best attempts to maintain a healthy looking skin.

So What Is Acne?

Human skin is covered in hundreds of thousands of microscopic hair follicles, often called pores, that connect to oil glands located under the skin. The glands are connected to the pores via small canals called follicles. A small hair grows through the follicle out of the skin. The oil glands secrete a thick oily liquid called sebum that

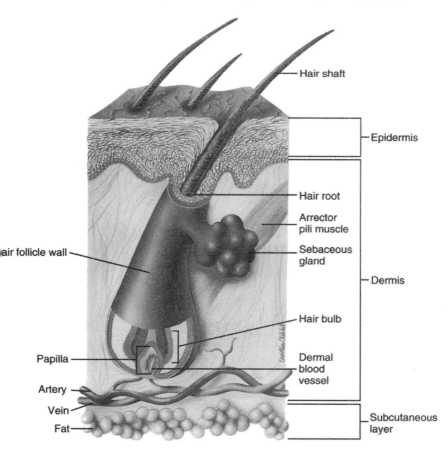

carries dead skin cells up the hair follicles and onto the surface of the skin as well as lubricates your hair and skin to keep it soft and smooth. These oil glands (also called sebaceous glands) are primarily located on the face, back, chest, shoulders, neck, and upper arms.

On our face and scalp skin we have an average of approximately 800 of these glands and follicles combined per square centimeter.

Most of the time, the sebaceous glands make the right amount of sebum. As a person approaches puberty (between the ages of ten and thirteen), the oil glands are stimulated by male hormones (androgens) produced by the adrenal glands of both males and females to make more sebum, and the glands often become overactive. Pores become clogged if there is too much sebum and too many dead skin cells. The secret to healthy skin is to control the oil production, not to dry out the oil completely as most treatments do.

Acne (*acne vulgaris*) is a skin disorder that involves an inflammatory condition of the oil glands at the base of hair follicles. It occurs when the pores in the skin are blocked, trapping the oil, dead skin, and bacteria in the hair follicles. The blocked oil oxidizes, causing an inflammation and an influx of white blood cells and resulting in a swelling and the formation of a blackhead. Meanwhile, normally present bacteria (Propionibacterium acnes) thrive in this excess oil. Immersed in excess oil, the bacteria can rapidly increase in number. As the bacteria multiply in a clogged pore, the pore becomes inflamed and white blood cells attack the bacteria. Pus forms as the lesion enters the whitehead stage. In more severe stages, an abscess—a pus-filled pocket within the skin—may form.

When you have just a few red spots, or pimples, you have a mild form of acne. Severe acne can include hundreds of pimples that can cover the face, neck, chest, and back. Or it can be bigger, solid red lumps or cysts that are painful.

Despite what you may have heard, acne is not contagious, and it is not caused by dirt.

Three Main Types of Acne

Noninflammatory Acne (mild)

Blackheads, also known as open comedones: These are said to be the first stage of acne. They are dilated or widened hair follicles that are filled with central, dark, solid plugs of sebum, dead cells, and bacteria, having undergone a chemical reaction resulting in the oxidation of melanin. The follicles are not completely blocked; the black appearance (can also be yellowish in color) is caused by oxidation, not dirt. You can't wash them away.

Whiteheads, also known as closed comedones: These form when skin cells and oil completely block the opening of a hair follicle. Since the air cannot reach the follicle, the material is not oxidized and remains white.

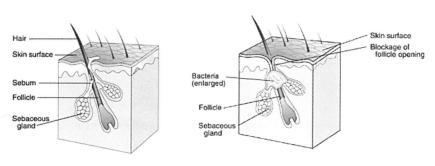

Normal follicle   Microcomedone

Inflammatory Acne (moderate)

A blackhead or whitehead can release its contents to the surface and heal or the follicle wall can rupture and inflammatory acne can ensue. This rupture can be caused by random occurrence or by picking or touching the skin. This is why it is important to leave acne prone skin relatively untouched.

Papules: This small, rough textured bump is a type of whitehead (5 mm or less) that occurs when the wall of a hair follicle breaks and caves in due to inflammation and infection. White blood cells rush in, and the pore becomes swollen, red, and has pus at the top.

Pustules: This whitehead is pus-filled and inflamed (the white blood cells have risen to the surface of the skin). Once they rupture into the skin, they form pustular heads and are what people usually refer to as a "zit" or "pimple."

Cystic Acne (severe)

A papule or pustule can completely collapse or explode, severely inflaming the surrounding skin and may engulf neighboring follicles. These lesions are called cysts or nodules.

Cysts: These sac-like lesions contain a buildup of white blood cells, bacteria, and dead cells in a liquid or semi-liquid state (boil-like infections). They can result in scarring and may be very painful and severely inflamed. Cysts and nodules often appear together to form nodulocystic acne, also very severe.

Nodules: Sometimes the bottom of a follicle will break off, which causes the follicle to completely collapse. This produces large solid, dome- or irregularly shaped, pus-filled lesions/lumps that extend deep into the skin, sometimes causing tissue damage and scarring if not treated. Nodular acne, which can be painful, is the most severe form of the disease.

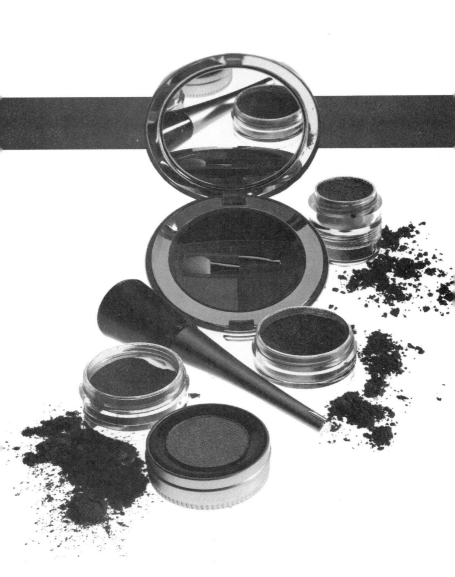

chapter 5
Factors That May Impact Acne

While it is one thing to understand what acne is, no one is exactly sure what causes these biological processes. Experts believe the primary cause is a rise in androgen levels—as noted previously, these are the hormones that significantly increase in boys and girls during puberty and cause the oil glands (sebaceous glands) to enlarge and make more sebum (oil) that triggers the series of events that result in acne breakouts. In men, the testosterone hormone originates in the male sexual organs, and in women, testosterone is produced in the ovaries and adrenal glands. After the testosterone is secreted into our body, it enters into our oil glands, where the enzyme 5-alpha-reductase converts the testosterone into the more potent androgen dihydrotestosterone (DHT).

Because 5-alpha-reductase is so responsive to hormone levels, it goes into overdrive when testosterone levels increase, causing an excess production of sebum.[39] Indeed, research indicates that the skin of acne patients shows a greater activity of 5-alpha-reductase in its conversion of testosterone to DHT.[40] This extra potent form of testosterone, DHT, is also one of the main reasons for acne flare-ups in and around intense workouts, because it skyrockets during workouts, especially during puberty. You don't necessarily want to stop this process completely, but supplementing before workouts with zinc and saw palmetto can help control the surge and reduce flare-ups.

Studies have also shown that even when lower levels of testosterone are present, the 5-alpha-reductase may increase its sensitivity to testosterone, triggering excess sebum production, for reasons that are not known.[41] While bewildering, it does at least tell us that rising hormone levels are not the sole trigger for escalating sebum production.

DHT is also an important contributor to other characteristics generally attributed to males, including muscular growth, facial and body hair growth, and deepening of the voice. It also seems to play a role in the development or exacerbation of benign prostatic hyperplasia and prostate cancer, though the exact reason for this is not known. So you can see that this process is a two-edged sword, both good and bad—you don't want to remove it, your body needs it, just control the excess amounts of it.

Here's the important point that I will continue to stress throughout this book: Contrary to what most acne treatments try to do, the secret to healthy skin is to control the oil production, not to dry out the oil. Your skin naturally produces oil because it needs it to function properly. Your natural oil helps lubricate as well as heal, protect, and moisturize your skin. Learning to work with your skin and oils, not against it, will help you tremendously.

> *Contrary to what most acne treatments try to do, the secret to healthy skin is to control the oil production, not to dry out the oil.*

Given that our goal is to control our oil production, it is worth noting that studies have shown zinc (an essential mineral that stimulates the activity of about 100 enzymes in the body) to inhibit the reductase enzyme, and zinc levels have been shown to be lower in patients with acne[42]; thus some doctors prescribe zinc supplement treatments to help increase the rate of acne treatment.[43] Also note that zinc is a common mineral deficiency, and especially so during the accelerated growth associated with puberty, which requires a boost of zinc. It is found in red meat, poultry, beans, nuts, seeds, seafood, whole grains, and dairy products and is a well-known antioxidant.

While not making any nutritional claims for zinc, cosmetically it has shown to help protect the skin from a variety of issues from sunburn to skin cancer. It also has been shown to absorb deeply into the skin and help protect it from the constant exposure to harmful external factors.

Stress

One of the most heavily researched as well as debated topics regarding acne is the role that stress plays in the formation of acne. Many studies have been able to find a direct link, especially in adults, between acne and stress, which comes in all shapes and sizes. There is emotional stress, such as a disagreement with a friend or grief over a loss. There are physical stresses, such as an illness or a lack of sleep or pushing our body to extremes. There are external stresses, such as climatic extremes and environmental toxins. Also there are internal stresses, such as anxiety about a speech or fear of punishment. Hormonal shifts and allergic responses are stresses. Relentless work pressure, financial worries, excessive caffeine, alcohol consumption, smoking, and unresolved traumas from the past—all of these are stresses that can exact a grim toll on our body and our psyche.

When your body is stressed, there is a hormone fluctuation that causes an increase in the amount of oil your skin secretes, which can cause acne to form or worsen. Since stress-induced acne looks identical to other forms of acne, the only indicator as to whether your acne was caused by stress is to keep track of acne breakouts. Was your last acne breakout around the time you had a major stressful event? If you can find a pattern between stressful events and breakouts, you may be predisposed to stress-induced acne. Try to reduce the stress in your life by using stress management techniques—positive attitude and self-talk, prayer and meditation, exercise, talking stressful situations out, breathing

> *When your body is stressed, there is a hormone fluctuation that causes an increase in the amount of oil your skin secretes, which can cause acne to form or worsen.*

and relaxation exercises, and especially SLEEP! All these will help you to be able to deal with stressful situations without letting them negatively impact you in any way, not just skin related.

From a scientific perspective, be aware that the mechanism of stress and acne is multifactorial. Stress and stressful eating habits elevate cortisol levels that raise one's blood sugar and provoke an insulin response, which increases body fat over time. Body fat can become the largest endocrine organ in the body that exacerbates the hormone problems, literally becoming an inflammation factory exponentially increasing the problem. Additionally, chronically elevated cortisol, blood sugar, and insulin dampens overall immunity and can lead to an autoimmune type response and promote inflammation that can lead to leaky gut syndrome, a condition where particles pass through the intestinal wall that should not, which can increase pathogenic bacteria in the gut. This condition can allow pathogenic bacteria to pass into the bloodstream and flow all over the body, including to the skin.

Hormonal Changes

Hormonal changes in women that occur around the menstrual cycle, pregnancy, and the use of synthetic birth control pills that mimic testosterone can affect sebum production. Also inappropriate metabolism of estrogen can lead to what is known as hydroxylated estrogen metabolites that promote inflammation.

Another major cause for the rise in androgen levels is covered in the following chapter, which covers basic nutrition and vitamins and minerals. It requires a full chapter of its own. The following are factors that can also trigger or aggravate an existing case of acne.

Exposure to Various Pollutants and Chemical Compounds

Exposure to various pollutants, such as tobacco smoke, grease and petroleum-based oils, coal tar derivatives, and chlorinated hydrocarbons, are also possible causes of acne, especially in industrial settings. Some of this can be avoided and some can't. The key is to eliminate the threats you have control over and give your body the right nutrition to maximize your personal immunity for the threats you cannot control. The easiest way to avoid certain pollutants is to not physically put them on, realizing that everything from makeup to sunscreen to perfumes and colognes contain chemicals that are very harmful to your skin and your body once they absorb into your bloodstream. Use organic products on your skin instead.

Acne can occur in response to bringing a variety of chemical compounds into one's body: corticosteroids (a class of chemicals often called steroid hormones and used in numerous anti-inflammatory drugs), halogens (chlorine, bromine, florine, astatine, and iodine), isonicotinic acid, diphenylhydantoin (an antiepileptic drug), and some psychotropics (chemical substances that cross the blood-brain barrier and act primarily upon the central nervous system where it affects brain function, including anxiolytics, euphoriants, stimulants, depressants, and hallucinogens).

Ninety percent of all the toxic exposure to poisons is in foods, personal care products, and even household goods and could be easily avoided by people simply *reading the ingredients* on product labels. Most people don't read labels because it's too much work or they don't understand what all the chemical terms really mean. But that's part of the secret: If the ingredients are full of chemicals, don't buy the product! Don't rub it on your skin and don't eat it!

Here are of some ingredients that you definitely want to avoid: BPA (bisphenol A), BPS (bisphenol S), phthalates, PFOA (perfluorinated chemicals), formaldehyde or formalin, parabens, dioxin, aluminum, flouride, benzophenones, toluene, quaternuim 15 & 51, TEA (triethanolamine), and PEG (polyethylene glycol). If you want to have more extensive information on the subject, I recommend a book called *Toxic Beauty* by Samuel S. Epstein, MD.

Elimination

Most modern diets don't include enough fiber for healthy bowel movements, which can lead to a toxic liver, overstressed kidneys, and skin problems. When the organs of elimination become imbalanced, the superficial circulation becomes filled with toxins, which clog the capillaries and lymphatic vessels that feed the sebaceous glands and cause inflammation and secondary infection. A buildup of toxins in your body causes acne.

Certain Cosmetics

Acne cosmetica, or acne caused by cosmetics, is a common mild form of acne. Cosmetic foundations, rouge, night creams, and

> *Cosmetic foundations, rouge, night creams, and moisturizers can worsen acne.*

moisturizers can worsen acne. Makeups that aren't organic, typically greasy cosmetics and facial creams, just clog your pores with the chemicals they are made of, blocking the flow that you need to create in order to keep the sebum buildup from happening. Acne cosmetica is small, rashy, pink bumps on the cheek, chin, and forehead. It develops over a period of a few weeks or months and persists for a long time. The outbreak can be stopped by ending the use of the particular cosmetic that triggers the onset.

Never buy cosmetic products that don't list their ingredients. Popular brand-name perfumes have even been found to contain *over 20 cancer-causing chemicals*, none of which are listed on the label. (Because it's a "proprietary secret"!)

If you go to the Environmental Working Group's Skin Deep cosmetic database (www.ewg.org/skindeep/), you can input the brand names of cosmetic and personal care items you use and get a toxicity report. You may be surprised by what you have been putting on your skin. Keep in mind that the government doesn't require health studies or pre-market testing of the chemicals in personal care products, even though just about everyone is exposed to them.

Over Washing and Aggressive Scrubbing

It shouldn't be a surprise that over washing, overly aggressive scrubbing, and repetitive touching or scratching can aggravate and worsen acne. It always seemed ironic to me that most acne treatments advise you to scrub their product in for a couple minutes to "remove dead skin cells," but this in turn aggravates the acne, causing more breakouts. Excessive cleansing with high detergent products can stimulate the oil glands, causing more congestion and pimples along with possibly dryness and irritation. The fact is that your skin is always shedding dead skin cells on its own, and there's no reason to force it. When you start to break out more, to wash the breakout spots more just continues to dry out your skin and washes away all the good oils that your body produces to keep it looking young and elastic.

Maintaining the Ideal pH

Our skin is made to naturally be our first line of defense against infection and the environment. The pH (potential of hydrogen) level of the skin refers to the balance of acid and alkaline. Within a scale from 1 being the most acidic to 14 being the most alkaline, 7 is considered a neutral reading for your skin's pH. Our skin has a thin, protective layer on the surface, often referred to as the acid mantle. This acid mantle, the combination of sebum (oil) and perspiration on the skin's surface, protects the skin and renders the skin less vulnerable to damage and attack by environmental factors such as the sun and wind and less prone to dehydration. Normal skin pH is somewhat acidic and in the range of 4.2 to 5.6. A healthy acid mantle inhibits the growth of foreign bacteria and fungi, and the skin remains healthier and has fewer blemishes. Acne, allergies, and other skin problems become more severe when the skin becomes more alkaline, thus maintaining the correct level of acidity is vital.

> *Acne, allergies, and other skin problems become more severe when the skin becomes more alkaline, thus maintaining the correct level of acidity is vital.*

The pH balance of the skin's acid mantle can be disrupted externally and internally by many factors. For instance, whatever contacts our skin (products, smoke, air, water, sun, pollution) can contribute to the breaking down of the acid mantle. Aging contributes to our skin becoming more acidic. And certainly our diet is significant in determining our internal and external pH levels. In the next chapter I emphasize *The Super Health Diet*, which consists of regularly alkalizing foods, such as leafy green vegetables, citrus fruits, tomatoes, carrots, etc., that will help keep your pH levels where they need to be.

The pH system works in 10-fold multiples, and each pH unit represents a 10-fold difference in alkalinity. For example, a soap with a pH of 10.5 has 10 times the alkalinity of a soap of pH 9.5. So-called "mild" soaps are often far too alkaline (pH 9.5–11) and remove the natural acid protection as well as extracting protective lipids (fats) from the skin. Irritated and eczematous skins tend to have a more alkaline pH, and washing with soap can increase this alkaline state and make the skin even more vulnerable to irritation and infection. Skin that is too alkaline can also be more susceptible to acne because a certain level of acidity is needed to inhibit bacterial growth on the skin. Choosing mild cleansers and toners that are slightly acidic (close to 5) will assist in properly maintaining the acid mantle and benefit all skin types. Note that a skin care product may claim to be pH balanced, but you can verify the actual pH of a product by using an at-home pH testing kit (available at most drugstores). A physician can also determine your skin's surface pH level and saliva tests can accurately indicate your body's overall pH level.

However, if you treat your skin with overly acidic products, such as alpha hydroxy acids, retinoic acid, beta hydroxy acids, and amino fruit acids, it can strip off the natural oils and weaken the skin's natural defenses to bacterial infection and environmental damage. If your skin starts to look dry or red, or if it becomes sensitive or breakouts increase, you may be using too strong of a product or applying it too often, so make sure you use products properly.

Topical antioxidants, such as vitamins A, C, E, and green tea, can be helpful in maintaining the acid mantle. First, they enrich the cells so that they can function optimally, and then they protect the cells from the previously mentioned environmental stresses and oxidation. For instance, vitamin C in the form of L-ascorbic acid is acidic by nature and formulations will have a low pH, so while not being considered a pH balancing antioxidant, they can be used safely and beneficially on the skin as long as it's not used at the same time as other acidic products. Sunscreen is another line of defense for the acid mantle as it shields the skin cells from sun damage and increases the skin's ability to protect itself, but a sunscreen is a potential carcinogen, so find a good one by going to www.ewg.org and reading their sunscreen report. Another problem with using sunscreens is that they block the natural production of vitamin D and necessitate the supplementation with vitamin D3.

So Daniel said to the steward whom the chief of the eunuchs had set over Daniel, Hananiah, Mishael, and Azariah, "Please test your servants for ten days, and let them give us vegetables to eat and water to drink. Then let our appearance be examined before you, and the appearance of the young men who eat the portion of the king's delicacies; and as you see fit, so deal with your servants." So he consented with them in this matter, and tested them ten days. And at the end of ten days their features appeared better and fatter in flesh than all the young men who ate the portion of the king's delicacies. Thus the steward took away their portion of delicacies and the wine that they were to drink, and gave them vegetables.

Daniel 1:11–16

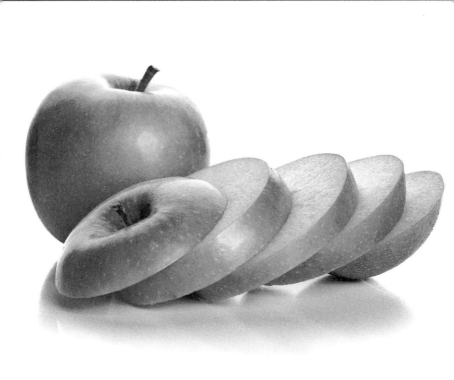

chapter 6

What You Eat and How You Supplement Really Does Matter

Despite the fact that many dermatologists and doctors still advise their patients that diet has little or even nothing to do with acne, the common-sense reality is that because your diet is intricately linked with the health of your entire being, this includes your skin health—whether it involves acne, premature wrinkles, or general skin clarity. A bad diet is definitely a cause for acne if for no other reason than it affects your hormones and gives you deficiencies in certain nutrients that are needed to regulate your hormones. It's the old adage: "You are what you eat." I believe that a bad diet is a primary cause for acne, though it isn't the sole cause.

> *Dermatologists and doctors should have been listening to their patients all along who were saying, "I ate a lot of junk food, then I broke out."*

The fact is that dermatologists and

doctors should have been listening to their patients all along who were saying, "I ate a lot of junk food, then I broke out." But rather than educate their teen and adult patients about lifestyle and diet choices that naturally help treat acne, many of the same dermatologists and doctors prescribe drugs that can have harmful long-term effects. Most of us, depending on sound advice from them, have been misled when it comes to acne and our diet and pay a price for it.

It is interesting that since the late 1800s, research has linked acne with diet, primarily related to sugar, fat, and chocolate. Old dermatology textbooks frequently recommended dietary restrictions as a form of treatment. And as early as 1931, researchers had discovered links between acne and carbs and impaired glucose tolerance (as some of the newer studies have documented as well). But during the 1960s, studies came out that disassociated diet with the formation of acne.

"This change occurred largely because of the results of two important research studies that are repeatedly cited in the literature and popular culture as evidence to refute the association between diet and acne," says Jennifer Burris, MS, RD, of the Department of Nutrition, Food Studies, and Public Health, Steinhardt School of Culture, Education, and Human Development, New York University. "More recently, dermatologists and registered dietitians have revisited the diet-acne relationship and become increasingly interested in the role of medical nutritional therapy in acne treatment."

In a 2013 paper published in the *Journal of the Academy of Nutrition and Dietetics*, Burris and her colleagues reviewed 27 studies on nutrition and acne.[44] Some of the more convincing evidence comes from a few recent studies of teenagers and young men (aged 15–25 years) who had acne. After the participants followed a low glycemic load diet, researchers documented decreases in inflammatory acne lesions. The glycemic load is how much a particular food will raise a person's blood sugar after eating it; basically, it is how much carbohydrate is in the food and how much each gram of the food raises blood sugar. The studies were small, but the findings were significant.

They concluded that a high glycemic index/glycemic load diet (typically sugary, processed foods) and possible frequent dairy consumption are the leading factors in establishing the link between diet and acne. So what explains this connection? Researchers say foods that spike blood sugar can also increase hormones. The hormones can stimulate oil production, which in turn, can trigger acne. "It's like a domino effect," said Burris. Makes sense, doesn't it?

I also want to note two other studies that you may find helpful and worth reading. One study found that people who drink two or more servings of dairy per day are 30 percent more likely to get acne.[45] Another study indicated that with a relatively minor change to a low glycemic diet, the reduction in acne was 50 percent.[46] Clearly, lifestyle choices play a role in the degree to which acne affects your skin.

Garbage In = Garbage Out

Whether for teens or adults, today's primary offender is a high sugar, empty carb, high trans fat content diet that increases blood sugar, causes abnormal development of the sebaceous glands, leading to acne. As noted previously, your blood sugar is directly tied to the delicate balance of hormones in your body. Surges in blood sugar trigger the androgen hormones to produce sebum in abundance that ultimately leads to acne breakouts.

> *Whether for teens or adults, today's primary offender is a high sugar, empty carb, high trans fat content diet that increases blood sugar, causes abnormal development of the sebaceous glands, leading to acne.*

What is a high trans fat content diet? Basically, it is today's teenage diet, which is high in carbohydrate-rich foods, such as bread, bagels, and chips, milk and cheese products. Think candy, sodas, corn and potato chips, french fries, cheeseburgers, hot dogs, and dairies. The combination of a diet that is high in sugar, refined carbohydrates, and trans fats but low in antioxidants leads to inflammation, oxidation, and stagnation that can manifest itself in your skin in the form of acne, rosacea, or premature aging.

As you will see, what is bad for your body is bad for your skin, so eating right to help clear up your skin is also helping every other aspect of your health.

I am about to go into a lot more detail for those of you who want the information, but to put it simply, "Garbage in equals garbage out." Your body is like a well-oiled machine, and if you give it the proper "oil," it will function perfectly. Our bodies, however, are far more advanced than any machine in that they have the ability to deal with the garbage we give it on a regular basis, but this compensation can cause a "hiccup" in other areas of health...acne being one of them. Prolonged "hiccups" will cause a crash if not corrected, and acne will be the least of your problems, so make sure to get this part under control.

A corollary problem to the wrong stuff that you are eating is the good food that you are not eating.

Here's just one example of how this works in your body. When you consume too much sugar, your body requires more chromium but your diet doesn't provide it, leading to a chromium deficiency. Researchers have found that people with unstable blood sugar levels have a high incidence of severe acne. High blood glucose has been linked as a causal agent of acne.[47] Chromium supplements have been demonstrated to boost the ability of the body to utilize glucose, which helps remove a source of energy for the bacteria that can accompany acne. High-chromium yeast has also been shown to improve glucose tolerance and enhance insulin sensitivity.[48]

Dietary Essential Nutrients

Before I go into detail, let me simplify nutrition for you.

Science has identified about 53 essential nutrients the human body must have in order to function at its peak. Since the body cannot produce a single one of these nutrients, each one must be obtained from food sources, dietary supplements, and exposure to sunshine. If we fall short, if we deprive our body of just one of these essential nutrients, we can suffer a breakdown in our health, resulting in dysfunction and disease that negatively affects our whole person. It's inescapable! All of your energies will be burned in trying to cope with the disease, and it will significantly limit all you wish to do as well as the person you'd like to be.

Think of it in these terms. If you were given a brand-new Lamborghini sports car that is designed to run on high-octane gasoline, would you even consider using regular low-grade fuel? How about diesel instead of gas? How about kerosene? No, of course not. Why? Because we know the result would be many thousands of dollars in repair bills. We would use only the manufacturer-specified gas and motor oil to not risk a catastrophe.

> *If you were given a brand-new Lamborghini sports car that is designed to run on high-octane gasoline, would you even consider using regular low-grade fuel?*

The same is true for the human body, which is far more complex and valuable than any fine sports car. It was designed to be fueled with clean high-octane fuel and to use high quality motor oil. Many of the foods we eat are like putting lighter fluid in our gas tank or putting used motor oil in our fine sports car. These foods during the short and long term can cause our bodies to sputter and misfire and lead to things from acne to disastrous consequences, such as major disease.

Beyond that, most people so overeat that it's as though they are filling their gas tank until it runs down the side of the car, then they roll down the back window and fill the back seat. The body has about as much capacity to deal with the constant over fueling as a car does with gas in the back seat.

Underscoring the nutrient problem is this conclusion of a report published online on August 11, 2010, in the *Journal of Nutrition*: "Nearly the entire U.S. population consumes a diet that is not on par with recommendations." Susan M. Krebs Smith and her colleagues at the National Cancer Institute evaluated data from 16,338 individuals aged two and older who participated in the 2001–2004 National Health and Nutrition Examination Survey (NHANES). With the exception of total grains, meat, and beans, the majority of the sample surveyed failed to consume the minimum recommendations for each of the USDA's food groups. I am no fan of the USDA's food groupings; however, it is important to note that almost all participants failed to consume enough dark green vegetables, orange vegetables, legumes, and whole grains. Total vegetable and milk recommendations were unmet by most people in more than half of the groups. Empty calories, including solid fats, added sugars, and alcoholic beverages were overconsumed by more than 90 percent of those aged 70 and younger. The authors of the study write, "This analysis indicates that nearly the entire U.S. population consumes a diet with fewer vegetables and whole grains than recommended, and that a large majority do not consume enough fruits, milk, and oils relative to recommendations. . . . A worrisome state in the context of the obesity epidemic and alarming rates of other diet-related chronic diseases."

According to a study published in the May 2008 edition of the *American Journal of Clinical Nutrition*, researchers at the University of Sydney discovered that a single serving of high glycemic/refined carbohydrates (e.g., table sugar, white bread, etc.) given to a lean, healthy young adult is enough to triple their inflammatory response to the surge in blood glucose. Acne is defined as an "inflammatory condition of the skin." Sugars and refined carbs definitely contribute to acne.

The Super Health Diet

I do not know of any diet that can come close to what my father, KC Craichy, has set forth in his book *The Super Health Diet*. There are more research studies that validate his Four Corners of Superfood Nutrition than any other nutritional approach in existence. It is a lifestyle approach that provides a comprehensive foundation for new levels of health awareness and life enhancement for everyone from elite athletes to the health challenged, who suffer from conditions such as diabetes, hypoglycemia, obesity, and eating disorders. What is unique about the Four Corners concept is that the individual four corners have been integrated into a single "unified theory" of nutrition science, including:

> *I do not know of any diet that can come close to what my father, KC Craichy, has set forth in his book The Super Health Diet.*

1. Eating fewer calories while maintaining optimal levels of all essential nutrients—Calorie Restriction with Optimal Nutrition, or CRON.

2. Eating and supplementing with generous amounts of broad-spectrum antioxidants.

3. Eating low glycemic impact foods and minimizing sugar.

4. Eating high quality foundational and fuel fats and supplementing with antioxidant essential fatty acids.

In my dad's book, he has a handy "At-a-Glance Foods to Eat and Foods to Avoid" that he graciously agreed to let me include for your health benefit:

Beverages

- Drink 8 to 12 glasses of spring or ionized structured micro-clustered water each day. I use spring water when I am out and use an Echo structured water system at home.

- Drink lightly caffeinated or caffeine-free organic herbal teas.

- Minimize fruit juices (except when mixed with high protein/fiber).

- Eliminate all soft drinks.

- Minimize coffee, alcoholic beverages, and artificial sweeteners.

Foods

- Eat a variety of salads, green vegetables, and bright colored, aboveground vegetables. Some good choices include broccoli, spinach, kale, mixed greens, asparagus, green beans, peppers, cucumbers, barley greens, radishes, garlic, and onions.

- Eat organic, free-range eggs.
- Eat berries (cranberries, strawberries, raspberries, and blueberries).
- Eat organic chicken, turkey, grass-fed beef and wild game, such as venison, buffalo, lamb, and deer.
- Eat antioxidant protected fish oil and certified mercury-free Pacific salmon, summer flounder, haddock, anchovies, and sardines. See www.vitalchoice.com.
- Use coconut oil, virgin olive oil, GLA, conjugated linolenic acid (CLA), and raw organic butter.
- Use Celtic Sea Salt or Real Salt brand mineral sea salts.
- Eat almonds, cashews, macadamia, and other nuts as well as organic coconut.
- Minimize all grains (bread, rice, and cereal), especially refined grains such as starches; avoid junk foods, pizza, and anything deep fried, such as french fries.
- Minimize pasteurized dairy products, such as milk, cheese, and cream.
- Minimize unfermented, genetically modified soy products.
- Minimize grain-fed commercial beef, pork products, and shellfish.
- Avoid farm-raised fish, such as catfish or salmon, and other fish with high mercury levels, such as tuna.

- Completely avoid hydrogenated oils found in processed foods, commercially prepared baked goods, margarines, and many snacks.

- Minimize all sugars (candy, cookies, cakes, and syrups) and chips.

The Super Health Diet is the last diet you will ever need! If you don't have the book, it is a must-read, so order your copy today at www.livingfuel.com.

Fats

Before I go too far into the biochemistry of fats, I want you to know that healthy fats are critical to life. The body is designed to manufacture most of the fats it needs. However, there are two major classes of fats the body needs but cannot manufacture on its own; hence they must be obtained through diet alone. These fats are the essential fatty acids.

The two essential fatty acids' classes are called omega-3 and omega-6 fatty acids. There are two categories of omega-3: plant sources, which contain the weaker omega-3 ALA, such as chia seed and flaxseed, and the more potent marine sources, such as salmon, tuna, mackerel, sardines, and anchovies, which contain the most effective forms of omega-3s—EPA and DHA. Scientists agree that only 10 to 15 percent of ALA converts to EPA in the body and about maybe 5 percent converts to DHA. Due to this poor conversion, plant omega-3, such as flaxseed, cannot on its own meet our body's nutritional requirement for EPA and DHA, so we must get them from marine sources—the best and most convenient method being to take antioxidant protected fish oils, such as my personal favorite Super-Essentials Omegas.

Also know that there is another fat known as "trans fat" that is essentially man-made. It was originally designed to replace butter as a fat that wouldn't go rancid. These are fats that the body cannot easily break down and promote inflammation by blocking the receptors that normally switch your metabolism on and off. The result is a vicious cycle of metabolic lethargy and increased insulin resistance. Most of the trans fats in the American diet are found in fried foods, shortening, margarine, donuts, partially hydrogenated oils, dressings, puffed cheese snacks, potato chips, tortilla chips, burgers, candies, and desserts. Finally, some healthy fats can convert to trans fats when exposed to high heat during cooking, especially frying. So let's look at where these fats come from and how they affect your body, especially in regards to possible effects on acne.

Most of the trans fats in the American diet are found in fried foods, shortening, margarine, donuts, partially hydrogenated oils, dressings, puffed cheese snacks, potato chips, tortilla chips, burgers, candies, and desserts.

Because the American diet is rich in omega-6 foods such as sesame, sunflower, corn, peanut, and soy, to name a few, and low in cold water fish, most people tend to eat far too much omega-6 and are dangerously deficient in omega-3. Both the level of omega-3 and the ratio of omega-6 to omega-3 fatty acids are critically important, and a healthy ratio of omega-6 to omega-3 fatty acids is thought to be approximately 3:1, and ideally 1:1. But many Americans have an imbalance of 20:1, which is theorized to cause all sorts of problems associated with modern life, including inflammatory diseases (with acne being one of them). It seems that omega-6 fatty acids are metabolized by the body in such a way as to increase pro-inflammatory chemicals. These chemicals appear to be intimately involved in the development of acne. For example, if you treat people experimentally with a chemical that blocks the activity of these chemicals, their acne improves.[49] The answer to this imbalance is usually as simple as taking fewer omega-6s and adding antioxidant protected fish oil to your diet. It has so many more health benefits than just helping with acne.

Omega-3 oils can also increase a useful molecule called *insulin-like growth factor binding protein-3*.[50] This chemical is like nature's sponge for soaking up IGF-1, which facilitates hormonal flare-ups of acne. So anything that helps regulate IGF-1 must be good, at least as far as acne is concerned. However, you don't want to eliminate IGF-1 as it also has benefits such as muscle and hair growth; you just want to control it. Trans fat is also metabolized into pro-inflammatory chemicals and needs to be avoided.[51]

High dose fish oil (equivalent to the oil in a serving of fatty fish) has been shown to have extraordinary health benefits, especially when taken along with antioxidants such as full-spectrum vitamin E, to-cotrienols, and tocopherols and the super antioxidant astaxanthin.

When GLA, the most powerful form of omega-6 found in borage seed oil and evening primrose oil, is combined with EPA from omega-3s, beneficial prostaglandins are produced.[52]

It is not good to cook with omega-3s, because when heated, they become trans fats. And you'll want to avoid using too much omega-6 as your cooking oil. So rely on olive, coconut, and palm oils as your all-around oils and don't deep fry.

Low Levels of Vitamin B5 (Pantothenic Acid)

This is detailed but extremely important, so stay with me. Vitamin B5 (pantothenic acid) is a major component of coenzyme A, which is necessary for hormone production as well as fatty acid metabolism, and is found in meat, whole grains, cereals, legumes, yogurt, and eggs and available as a supplement. In 1995, the journal *Medical Hypotheses* printed a hypothesis by Dr. Lit-Hung Leung that attempted to link low levels of vitamin B5 with acne formation.[53] He noted that as hormone production increases during puberty, the body chooses to use coenzyme A to produce hormones and neglects fatty acid metabolism. Because the body uses coenzyme A for hormone production instead of fatty acid metabolism, sebum (oil) levels rise and acne follows. Supplementing with megadoses of vitamin B5 or applying topical creams allows for enough circulating B5 to address both bodily processes, thus helping clear up acne.[54]

> *Supplementing with megadoses of vitamin B5 or applying topical creams allows for enough circulating B5 to address both bodily processes, thus helping clear up acne.*

Dr. Leung gave his acne patients huge doses of vitamin B5, from 1 to 20 grams, that helped clear the acne, but caused some gastrointestinal gas and bloating. Other than that, no adverse side effects were noted. Considering the biochemical pathways involved, to reduce the B5 dosage to a more reasonable level it has been suggested that L-Carnitine be added, because it transports fatty acids across the mitochondrial membrane where they can be oxidized. Using the modified protocol with pantethine 750 mg with 250 mg of L-Carnitine three times a day has shown excellent success rates in minimizing acne.

While Dr. Leung's research is exciting and fascinating, no legal claims regarding his findings or the modified protocol, have been fully proven yet. However, it is exciting when you consider this information along with the fact that B5 has been shown to be an effective nutrient cosmetically for "skin conditioning." And that it helps the body to maintain the skin in good condition, affixes the skin, smoothes the skin, affixes connective tissue, helps wound healing, protects from free radicals, and helps cell renewal when applied cosmetically.[55] Regardless of how you look at it, vitamin B5 is just plain good for your skin—acne or no acne.

Regarding carnitine, it has cosmetically been shown to be cleansing, helps to enhance stability, helps to keep the body surface clean when applied cosmetically, and has been shown to enhance the action of the B5, allowing you to take less B5 than the dosages that studies have suggested, and transports storage fat and even serves as a natural cellulite ingredient.[56]

Other Vitamins

Vitamins are catalysts that enable other nutrients to work in our bodies. They are important life-supporting organic materials that are not generally constructed in the human organism and therefore should be taken as such in the form of their provitamins in food. The split of vitamins into fat-soluble (A, D, E, K) and water-soluble (B and C) vitamins allows the inclusion of their origin in different foodstuffs.

The majority of people eat far less vegetables than the recommended amount. Vegetables are the main source of vitamins in your diet if you are not taking vitamin supplements. You either have to eat more vegetables or start taking vitamin supplements. It's just as simple as that.

Most of the known vitamins are indispensable for the health of the skin and hair. It is important to take a complete and high quality multivitamin with minerals as a simple way of getting most of the basic nutrients the body requires. Avoid synthetic vitamins. It can also be beneficial to regularly take a balanced "stress" B-complex with meals, which improves cellular oxygenation and energy.

> *Most of the known vitamins are indispensable for the health of the skin and hair.*

Vitamins can also show a good effect when used on the skin surface and are added to many cosmetic products. Some of the most important components for cosmetics are vitamin A with the precursor beta carotene, vitamin E, and the B vitamins, and especially biotin.

As the supporting pillar for our body's entire immune system, our skin's defensive cells against disease-causing agents must always be ready, for which vitamin C is primary and well established through research for its positive effects. On the cosmetic side, vitamin C has been shown to affix the skin, help smooth the skin, help wound healing, affix connective tissue, and is said to help protect from free radicals, help cell renewal, and offer a good percutaneous absorption and decompose there into free vitamin C. Vitamin C is used cosmetically in whitening, anti-aging, and acne products.[57]

Studies have shown a strong relationship between a decline in the levels of the well-known antioxidants vitamin A and E and an increase in the severity of acne. Patients with severe acne had significantly lower plasma concentrations of vitamins A and E than did those with lower acne grade and the age-matched healthy controls. Administration of vitamin A and E to patients with acne was shown to improve their acne condition.[58]

To detail that a bit more, realize that vitamins A and E protect the skin's cell membrane against free radicals that can attack the cells and through this weaken the immune system. When these vitamins are diminished, the skin's protective cells begin to calcify and stop the production of defensive materials. Vitamin A in its pure form (retinol) and the derivate beta carotene (which builds vitamin A itself in the body) stimulate cell renewal and help smooth the skin. It gives tired cells a push to regularly divide. Through this, growing young cells are encouraged, which makes the skin more resistant and vital. Beta carotene is also the best internal skin protectant against sunlight. The highly important (for the skin) vitamin A can be found mostly in dark leafy vegetables as well as egg yolks, tomatoes, and oranges.

On the cosmetic side, I want to also mention four other vitamins for their values as cosmetic ingredients. Niacin (vitamin B3), which can make the skin uncomfortably flush by increasing blood flow, has been shown to be a wonderful antistatic and smoothing. It has also been shown to seek to achieve an even skin surface by decreasing roughness or irregularities, promoting circulation, expanding blood vessels, and affixing the skin and connective tissue. It also helps cell renewal. Niacin is used in anti-cellulite products and for raw, reddened, and impacted skin.[59]

Niacinamide (vitamin B3) is a flush-free form of niacin and has also been shown to be smoothing and have the same benefits as niacin.

Turmeric is another ingredient that helps stimulate blood flow and overall health in general.

Pyridoxine (vitamin B6) has been shown to be skin conditioning and helps to maintain the skin in good condition, has a sebostastic and balancing effect, and helps wound healing.[60] A lack of vitamin B6 leads to neuritis and seborrhoea dermatitis. If it is used directly on the skin, it can help regulate sebum production. It is therefore used in products against oily, impure skin, mixed skin and acne.[61]

Anti-inflammatories and Antioxidants

Because acne is an inflammatory condition of the skin, it makes sense that one way to battle inflammation is with anti-inflammatories. For instance, our skin and sebum are constantly exposed to oxidative stress (UV rays from overexposure to the sun, ozone in smog, chemicals in personal care products) and requires antioxidant protection. Without that protection, free radicals cause oxidative damage to sebum, which lowers the oxygen content in sebum and leads to changes in sebum that make it a more suitable environment to P. Acnes bacteria. Bacteria then multiply in the hair follicles and further increase inflammatory damage, leading to the angry, red pimples we hate.

Research has shown that people with acne have significantly lower levels of several antioxidant nutrients compared to people with healthy skin. Similarly, studies show that people with acne have higher levels of inflammatory chemicals in the blood. Acne patients are under significant systemic inflammation and oxidative stress, and their antioxidant defense cannot cope with the load.

> *Research has shown that people with acne have significantly lower levels of several antioxidant nutrients compared to people with healthy skin.*

Managing inflammation and correcting antioxidant depletion is one of the keys to getting over acne. This can be done primarily through proper diet and lifestyle changes. If you implement *The Super Health Diet* as mentioned previously, you will find that its Four Corners of Superfood Nutrition is low sugar, low glycemic, and loaded with a broad spectrum of antioxidants that help regulate and quench the destructive fire of oxidation and inflammation.

Sugar is the greatest inflammatory substance in our diet, but trans fats are not far behind them. Trans fats promote inflammation by blocking the receptors that normally switch your metabolism on and off.

Vitamin E is among the most important antioxidants in the skin, and studies have shown that it can protect sebum from oxidative damage. The topical application of vitamin E should be on the to-do list for anyone with acne.

Glycation

Beyond antioxidants, another new front line of preventing damaged skin is anti-glycation agents. Glycation involves the complex process of cross-linking of sugars with amino acids that alters the structure and function of proteins. Basically, it is a useless, caramelized protein. Glycated proteins are less elastic and more rigid than normal proteins, thus producing findings from decreased contractility in the heart to decreased skin rebound.

There are two primary sources for glycation. The first source is the food we eat. The browning of food is a cooking technique that helps to give desirable flavor to food. It is achieved by heating or cooking sugars with proteins in the absence of water, and in this process Advanced Glycation End products, or AGEs, are formed. Since grains, vegetables, fruits, and meat all have proteins, this browning effect is an indication of AGEs. It is estimated that 30 percent of food-borne AGEs are absorbed when ingested.

The second source for AGEs happens inside your body through normal metabolism and aging. Carbohydrates, either simple or complex, are absorbed by your body to affect your blood sugar levels. Most of your blood sugar goes to providing the energy your body needs to properly function. However, a small proportion of your blood sugar binds to proteins in your blood and creates AGEs.

Cooked foods and sugar are the primary contributors to glycation. Implementing *The Super Health Diet* will go a long way in your fight against glycation. I recommend eating at least one half of your diet as uncooked or minimally cooked live foods, such as salads and vegetables mostly. While it may be impossible to totally avoid foods cooked at high temperatures, it is possible to reduce exposure by changing the way food is prepared. Consider steaming, boiling, poaching, stewing, stir-frying, or using a slow cooker. These methods not only cook foods with a lower amount of heat, but they create more moisture during the cooking process. Water or moisture can help delay the browning reaction associated with higher temperature cooking. Marinating foods in olive oil, cider vinegar, garlic, mustard, lemon juice, and dry wines can also help.

I recommend eating at least one half of your diet as uncooked or minimally cooked live foods, such as salads and vegetables mostly.

In 2006, the American Academy of Dermatology sponsored three studies to investigate other uses for glucosamine. Alexa Kimball of Harvard led one of these studies and reported that her findings indicated that glucosamine could possibly treat skin damage caused from ultraviolet radiation.[62] Their findings also demonstrated that glucosamine can accelerate the speed in which a skin wound or cut heals, increases the hydration of skin, and decreases wrinkles. Glucosamine is able to do this because it is a building block of connective tissue, and it stimulates the production of hyaluronic acid (one of the three major components of the dermis layer of your skin) that leads to its remarkable power to help rebuild skin tissue as well as cartilage found in joints and helps your skin hold on to water, which gives skin fullness and radiance and is associated with a youthful appearance.

Although "glycation" is not mentioned in this study, it talks about using different nutrients to restore elasticity and hydration, both of which tie into glycation. The good news is that if glucosamine can stimulate production of hyaluronic acid in your joints, it can likely do the same for your skin! One of your goals should be to restore the hyaluronic acid that will make your skin plumper, more youthful looking, and better hydrated.

Hyaluronic acid's cosmetic value is that of an antistatic, humectant, skin conditioning, and moisturizing. Its cosmetic characteristics are that it increases the water content of the skin and helps keep it soft and smooth, maintains the skin in good condition, holds and retains moisture, and has a skin tightening effect.[63] Because it exists in human connective tissue, hyaluronic acid can bind a large amount of water and be stored in the connective tissue matrix, which gives the skin a smooth and full appearance.[64] It builds a film on the skin that fixates moisture, effective on the skin surface so that the smoothing effect is left if hyaluronic acid products are taken away.[65] Even one percent aqueous solutions of hyaluronic acid form a viscoelastic network through intermolecular clustering that binds the water extremely tightly. Hyaluronic acid is therefore recommendable as a moisturizer for skin care, because it forms an invisible, air-permeable film that protects the dermis from dehydration even at low relative humidity. Hyaluronic acid is nontoxic, nonallergenic, and nonirritating.[66]

Nature is doing her best each moment to make us well. She exists for no other end. Do not resist. With the least inclination to be well, we should not be sick.

Henry David Thoreau

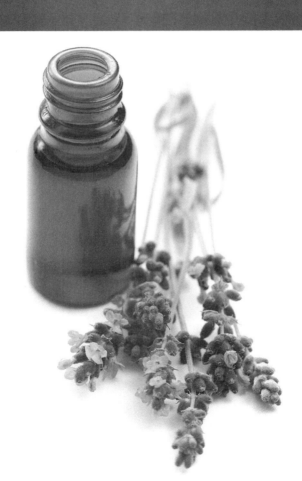

chapter 7

Is "Oil Free" the Correct Method?

As was demonstrated in the history section, for centuries people have been drying out their skin to remove acne, and it is still the goal of most of the popular acne treatments used today. Sulfurs have been used since the Romans, benzoyl peroxide since the 1920s, Retin A since the 1960s, Accutane and its knockoffs since the 1980s, and salicylic acid all with the same goal: Dry out the problem areas. And to a certain extent, it makes sense. "Acne," we're told over and over, "is caused by an excess in oil buildup, so remove the oils."

But what so often is forgotten or overlooked in this approach is that your skin produces this oil for a reason. It needs its natural oils to be healthy in the same way your mouth needs saliva, your eyes need tears, and so on. Your skin's natural oil is essential to skin health and even helps to clear acne.

Your skin's natural oil is essential to skin health and even helps to clear acne.

When a company advertises their products as "oil free," what they mean is that there is no oil in the product and not necessarily that the product removes the oils, though most of them do. They do this because of the fear of putting more oils on your face, even though many are helpful.

So is putting "oil free" products that completely dry the oils from your face the correct thing to do?

Is it wise to remove the oils that give you the moist, smooth, healthy looking skin you want, and then end up with dry, red, peeling, unhealthy looking skin, as well as prematurely age your skin?

Is this method simply treating the symptom rather than getting to the cause of acne?

Wouldn't it be better to control the oils and nourish the skin rather than remove them?

My Questions Regarding "Oil Free"

Step back for a moment and reflect on what I experienced in my search for something, anything that would help me with my acne condition. Most of the acne products I used were advertised as "oil free," and even when I went to the most popular acne brand's website, it warned me of all the dryness I would have as a result of their treatment. One of the top three acne products even encourages their users to purchase "humidifiers for your rooms and extra moisturizing creams," because they will be so dry from the treatment. Yet they turn around and say that "there is no such thing as too much moisture"! If their "drying out" concept is valid, why the glaring inconsistency?

Besides being straight chemicals and incredibly drying, all of the popular products I tried raised a lot of questions. For instance, they were all multistep processes: "Rub the exfoliator in for thirty seconds, wash it off, let the main drying product sit on your skin for two minutes, then wash it off and moisturize," etc. Why do we dry out our whole face to remove all the much-needed oils from our whole face, including the already clear parts, just to get the pimples?

Another question I had was the basic approach of how one should take care of your skin, which is the largest organ of your body. To use products that strip the oil out of our skin leaves it to trying to repair itself by replacing the oil stripped away, with the inevitable result being a cycle of being tight and dry followed by an oil slick. Each time we strip the oil away, our skin overcompensates for the lack of moisture by creating more oil. Dry, irritated skin is followed by oily skin that traps debris and becomes inflamed. How does that not lead to an endless cycle of breakouts?

> *Each time we strip the oil away, our skin overcompensates for the lack of moisture by creating more oil.*

Benzoyl peroxide and salicylic acid are the two most common active ingredients in acne medications that are primarily used as skin drying agents. If skin drying were the key to solving acne, these two compounds would have ended the acne epidemic long ago.

In researching these ingredients, the most obvious place to start is what the name means. Basic high school chemistry would tell you that peroxide is by nature an oxidant that causes inflammation and is hyper-aging to the skin. As I mention elsewhere in this book, what we want on our skin is antioxidant and anti-inflammatory.

So does putting on a solution that is drying, oxidizing, and inflammatory sound like something good for acne? Not to me it doesn't. People have had success with treatments using this by drying their skin until the condition resolves itself, but using a compound that dries, inflames, and ages is far from ideal. I've tried the products that use these ingredients, and I can tell you as well as virtually every other person I have talked to about this, it really is not a pleasant experience. Your skin is so unnaturally dry that you feel as though your face is going to crack, and then there are the potential long-term skin issues associated with harsh chemicals. I reiterate that it is *not* natural or advisable to deplete your skin of natural oils and then attempt to replete them with unnatural moisturizers. There's a better way.

Salicylic acid, used correctly, can be effective. Unfortunately, virtually all products that use this compound try to use it as a drying agent similar to benzoyl peroxide, which results in most of the same problems. Salicylic acid, however, comes from the "aspirin" family, which is a well-known anti-inflammatory and not an oxidant. So if one could use this compound in conjunction with natural oils, antioxidants, and other skin nutrients, it would be a powerful tool against acne—essentially moisturizing and drying at the same time, while providing anti-inflammatory and antioxidant and other skin-nourishing benefits.

The right approach will be anti-inflammatory, antioxidant, and nourish the skin.

The Frightening Reality of Drug Absorption

Our skin "drinks" or absorbs everything we put on it topically, whether it includes vitamins and minerals or toxins and chemicals. Any chemical that is combined with the active ingredients that are in all the popular treatments will be absorbed into your bloodstream and circulated around the body, causing all kinds of problems. That's certainly the case with chemicals in all personal care products, from makeups to moisturizers to perfumes to acne products. And nothing I found in the acne products I tried was anything but acids and chemicals and preservatives that are toxic to the body.

> *Your body wasn't designed to have its oils removed nor was it designed to handle these unnatural substances internally or externally.*

Your body wasn't designed to have its oils removed nor was it designed to handle these unnatural substances internally or externally. So what are the consequences—both short- and long-term—for using all those drugs, chemicals, and oil-removing scrubs on your skin? As a result of all these added chemicals, on top of the exhaustion of the oil glands from overproducing and removing oils, we are going to see an increase of premature aging of the skin in this generation on top of a host of internal issues from repeated application and absorption. Your skin and body doesn't know what to do with these, and we don't even know all the side effects that will happen later in life as a result of using these products.

For instance, a 2008 Environmental Working Group study revealed the presence of 16 chemicals from 4 chemical families in the bodies of 20 American girls aged 14 to 19. Chemicals from these families, phthalates, triclosan, musks, and parabens, are all commonly used in cosmetics and body care products and are capable of disrupting the hormone system according to laboratory tests.[67] Emerging research suggests that teens may be particularly sensitive to exposures to hormone-disrupting chemicals, given the complex hormonal signals that guide the rapid growth and development of the reproductive system, the brain, and the bone, blood, and immune systems during adolescence.[68]

That is frightening! Don't add gas to the fire by continuing to use these products on your skin.

Work with Your Skin, Not Against It

The question I want to ask you is, why does our skin naturally produce oil? And the simple answer was, because it needs it. It helps lubricate, heal, protect, and moisturize your skin so that it functions properly, leading to skin that is clear, beautiful, and glowing. Oil alone will not bring you acne. It is not an evil force to be driven away; it is naturally occurring and there for the benefit of your skin.

The key to achieve healthy skin is to keep the moisture of your natural oils but prevent the oils from clogging the pores. You aren't looking for a product to remove the oils from your skin, which makes your skin dry and unhealthy looking. Rather, you need to work with your skin, not against it, and reduce the amount of oil it is producing, which makes all the difference in the world, particularly during periods of hormonal changes. And you control it not by drying it out, but by giving your skin the nutrients it needs to be healthy, both internally and externally.

I began to research the best natural ingredients for acne and the skin for both internal and external application and then tried combinations of them to make my own homemade solution. I found that when you give your skin a combination of vitamins, antioxidants, fatty acids, phytonutrients, and essential oils, it works miracles on your skin. For instance, I found that vitamin A applied on its own isn't as effective as applying a combination of it with vitamins E and C, some aloe, and an essential oil as well as green tea extract, because all of these ingredients are needed by the skin. When your skin gets what it needs, it basically will heal itself.

> *I found that when you give your skin a combination of vitamins, antioxidants, fatty acids, phytonutrients, and essential oils, it works miracles on your skin.*

Drugs work the opposite way. All drugs have side effects, and one must always weigh whether the side effects are worse than the original condition. If you take multiple drugs at a time, you combine the side effects of them, and the reaction of them together adds a whole host of different side effects not listed on the warnings for the drugs individually. In fact, research now suggests that if you are taking five or more drugs, it is clinically impossible to predict the side effects.

By way of contrast, when you combine nutrients, you can't yet predict all the benefits. They are too numerous, as is true of what I discovered with essential oils.

Essential Oils

Essential oils are gentle and inexpensive tools that help keep your skin from overcompensating in oil production and clear outbreaks as well as promote healing of acne scars. Essential oils are well-known for their antiseptic, antibacterial, and calming properties.

Although therapeutic grade essential oils are more expensive, I recommend choosing them. Cheaper oils may be adulterated and worsen acne problems. Lemon, geranium, palmarosa, and petit-grain are essential oils that help to regulate the control of sebum. Other useful oils include juniper, lavender, lime, neroli, rosemary, and sandalwood.

Tea Tree Oil

Tea tree oil, commonly referred to as *melaleuca*, has long been used to work wonders with practically all viral, bacterial, and fungal infections, and especially with health conditions affecting the skin. I found it effective in helping to treat my skin problems, such as oily skin, blisters, and acne.

In fact, a 1990 comparative study of 5 percent tea tree oil versus 5 percent benzoyl peroxide in the treatment of acne showed a significant reduction in inflamed and noninflamed lesions when applied topically.[69] Although tea tree oil may initially take a little longer to see positive effects, once it kicks in, it has been shown to be on par with benzoyl peroxide. But more importantly, it will limit the side effects that you can get from benzoyl peroxide, such as irritations, rashes, burning sensations, or dryness.

> *Although tea tree oil may initially take a little longer to see positive effects, once it kicks in, it is on par with benzoyl peroxide.*

A 2010 study at Sweden's Skane University Hospital also showed that tea tree oil was able to reduce allergic contact dermatitis by 40.5 percent, showing it to be effective in helping to treat eczema and at the very least it is superior to zinc oxide or cobestasone butyrate.[70]

While there are impressive benefits suggested in the research for the use of tea tree oil for the treatment of acne, it has not yet resulted in approved nutritional claims. What has been approved are certain cosmetic claims (INCI function), including that it is antimicrobial, with the characteristics of reducing the activity of microorganisms on the skin and has antimicrobial properties.[71]

Another reference notes it is fungicidal, helps oily skin, and extends shelf life in cosmetics. It is said to have very strong antimicrobial and fungicidal properties.[72]

Lavender Oil

Lavender is a mild but potent essential oil made by processing the flowers of Lavandula augustafolia, an evergreen plant that is native to the Mediterranean. It has antiseptic, anti-inflammatory, and analgesic properties that have a balancing effect on the skin, helps scar tissue to heal, and can generally be used for all skin types. It absorbs quickly to contain the infection and reduce the pain. Lavender oil is one of the few oils that can be applied directly to the skin. Try mixing 5 drops of lavender oil and 15 drops of sweet almond oil to make a soothing serum for the skin. Lavender oil is commonly used as a burn salve and as a natural cleanser for skin cuts and abrasions as well. It contains properties that help accelerate the wound healing process, meaning it may also help accelerate the healing of existing acne lesions.

There is very significant research that suggests lavender oil is also effective in treating acne, but no nutritional claims have been approved to make. However, the approved cosmetic claims (INCI function) is that it works as a tonic and has masking benefits. Characteristically, it produces a feeling of well-being on skin, calms the skin, and has a cell renewing effect.[73]

Bergamot Oil

The oil from the peel of the bergamot fruit has an antiseptic action and ability to promote skin growth that makes it another valuable tool for treating acne. Its antibacterial action helps to kill the bacteria on the skin before it can react to create blackheads and pimples. Bergamot has an added property of helping to control excess oil production in

The oil from the peel of the bergamot fruit has an antiseptic action and ability to promote skin growth that makes it another valuable tool for treating acne.

the skin, attacking acne from two sides.

The approved cosmetic claim of bergamot oil is that it has masking benefits with the characteristics of being antiseptic and deodorizing.[74]

Despite the best of efforts, many people develop acne scars, which can be incredibly difficult to accept or to live with. However, it is important to keep in mind that this process is a significant part of the skin's natural recovery and that there are several different acne scar treatment solutions available, which will be able to minimize the appearance of unsightly scars.

The more severe the type of acne you have suffered from, the more serious the extent of acne scarring will be. White and blackheads are noninflammatory, quite superficial, and usually heal without any scarring. However, types such as cystic acne extend deep into the dermis and their development involves inflammation, infection, and significantly more damage to the dermis. Fortunately, there are a variety of treatments available to lessen the appearance of this damage, including home remedies for acne scars. There are two that I found to be helpful.

Aloe Vera or Aloe Barbadensis Extract

Because of its powerful astringent, anti-inflammatory, antibacterial, and antiseptic properties, aloe vera gel has long been used to treat wounds[75] and burns and is highly acclaimed for its health, beauty, medicinal, and skin care properties. The juice extracted from the leaves of the plant contains a vast range of vitamins, minerals, amino acids, and enzymes that make it a natural acne scar treatment. It is best used in its purely natural form and applied directly onto the scars. To further enhance or broaden its benefits, there are several natural ingredients that could be added to it either to accelerate the healing process or to lighten the affected area.

There are no nutritional claims for aloe vera, but the evidence is staggering. The approved cosmetic claims (INCI function) of aloe vera is that it is an emollient with the characteristics of softening and smoothing the skin, giving moisture, healing wounds, preventing infections, and promoting self-healing with sunburns. It also has a cooling effect, helping to protect against skin irritation, and it provides a slight UV protection.[76]

Rose Hip Oil

Rose hip oil (of the rosaceae family) is a cold pressed oil that is extracted from the seeds of a wild rose bush, and because of its powerful nutritional composition and antimicrobial and balancing properties, it is a valuable tool in the healing of acne scars as well as scarring caused by eczema, scarring from psoriasis, stretch marks due to pregnancy or sudden weight gain, wrinkles, hyper-pigmentation caused by aging or uneven skin tone. Rose hip oil contains

80 percent essential fatty acids (very high in vitamins A, C, and E). Linoleic and linolenic, also known as omega-6 and omega-3, are important nutrients for producing healthy skin, especially in the case of repairing the membranes. Regenerating the skin is one way of healing scars from acne. You can apply this oil directly to the skin after each time you cleanse. You will be surprised about the difference this oil can make!

Once again, the approved cosmetic function (INCI function) of the cosmetic ingredient rose hip oil is that it is masking and is a tonic with the characteristics being that it produces a feeling of well-being on skin and hair.[77] No nutritional claims have been approved.

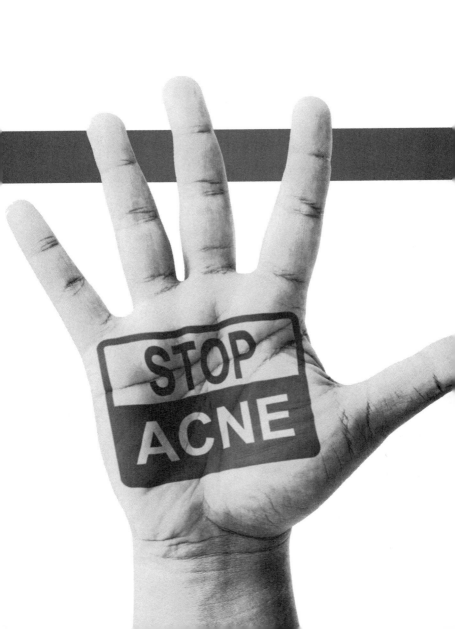

chapter 8

Accutane and Its Knockoff Brands

Accutane (also known as isotretinoin, Roaccutane, Amnesteem, Claravis, and Isotroin) is a powerful drug that was discovered in 1979 when it was first given to patients with severe cystic acne, most of whom reacted with dramatic clearing of their acne symptoms. It is a vitamin A derivative (13-cis-retinoic acid) that is administered orally in pill form with a meal that contains an adequate amount of fat, normally for a period 15 to 20 weeks,[78] although it is also sometimes prescribed at lower dosages for up to six months or longer. It was originally prescribed as the "nuclear option" for acne for people who do not respond to topical applications such as benzoyl peroxide and other standard antibiotic treatments,[79] but has gained in popularity in the past 25 years and is prescribed more and more frequently for less severe acne.[80] This practice is controversial, because Accutane is a serious medication that can cause long-lasting side effects.

Exactly how Accutane works on a cellular level is unknown, but it affects all four ways that acne develops. It dramatically reduces the size of the skin's oil glands (35 to 58 percent) and even more dramatically reduces the amount of oil these glands produce (around 80 percent).[81] Acne bacteria (P. acnes) live in skin oil. Since oil is dramatically reduced, so is the amount of acne bacteria in the skin.[82] And it slows down how fast the skin produces skin cells inside the pore, which helps pores from becoming clogged in the first place.[83]

After coming on the market, the dramatic results of Accutane propelled it to quickly become a highest-selling prescription drug. It has been shown to achieve partial or complete clearance of acne in about 95 percent of people who complete a cycle, regardless of whether they have inflammatory or noninflammatory acne,[84] and the majority experience long-term remission of acne symptoms.

Impressive, yes, but even while it was hailed as the breakthrough treatment for patients with severe acne, dangerous side effects have affected thousands and thousands of users since then. In the summer of 2009, Accutane manufacturer Roche Pharmaceuticals recalled the drug from American drugstores and also in several other countries after juries had awarded millions of dollars in damages to former Accutane users over inflammatory bowel disease claims (Crohn's disease and ulcerative colitis). You can only find the knockoff brands now, which have many of the same detrimental effects.

In the summer of 2009, Accutane manufacturer Roche Pharmaceuticals recalled the drug from American drugstores.

So what are the side effects? According to the Food and Drug Administration Accutane Medication Guide, these are possible side effects, but there are other numerous serious warnings about how Accutane should and should not be used[85]:

- Can cause birth defects (deformed babies), loss of a baby before birth (miscarriage), death of the baby, and early (premature) births.

- May cause serious mental health problems (depression, psychosis, and suicide).

- Serious brain problems. Accutane can increase the pressure in your brain. This can lead to permanent loss of eyesight and, in rare cases, death. Stop taking Accutane and call your doctor right away if you get any of these signs of increased brain pressure: bad headache, blurred vision, dizziness, nausea or vomiting, seizures (convulsions), and stroke.

- Stomach area (abdomen) problems. Certain symptoms may mean that your internal organs are being damaged. These organs include the liver, pancreas, bowel (intestines), and esophagus (connection between mouth and stomach). If your organs are damaged, they may not get better even after you stop taking Accutane.

- Bone and muscle problems. Accutane may affect bones, muscles, and ligaments and cause pain in your joints or muscles. Accutane may stop long bone growth in teenagers who are still growing.

- Skin problems—rashes, red or inflamed eyes, blisters on legs, arms, or face and/or sores in your mouth, throat, nose, eyes, or if your skin begins to peel.

- Hearing problems. Your hearing loss may be permanent.

- Vision problems. Accutane may affect your ability to see in the dark. This condition usually clears up after you stop taking Accutane, but it may be permanent. Other serious eye effects can occur. If you wear contact lenses, you may have trouble wearing them while taking Accutane and after treatment.

- Lipid (fats and cholesterol in blood) problems. Accutane can raise the level of fats and cholesterol in your blood. This can be a serious problem.

- Serious allergic reactions, such as hives, a swollen face or mouth, or have trouble breathing.

- Blood sugar problems. Accutane may cause blood sugar problems including diabetes.

- Decreased red and white blood cells. Call your doctor if you have trouble breathing, faint, or feel weak.

- Accutane may damage the digestive system and, for example, cause ulcerative colitis.

- Accutane may create blood clots that obstruct blood flow and may lead to heart attacks.

- Common, less serious side effects of Accutane include dry skin, chapped lips, dry eyes, drying of nose, and nose bleeding.

I did not make this list up to frighten you away from it. This is directly from the FDA website.

I did not make this list up to frighten you away from it. This is directly from the FDA website. Here's another interesting fact. Isotretinoin, the active ingredient in Accutane, was originally developed as a chemotherapy drug, and it's still used as that. During the chemotherapy trials, doctors noticed patients' acne clearing. So while Accutane was initially meant as a chemotherapy drug, which does serious damage to the body, they found that it also helps acne. Should it surprise us that it has such frightening side effects?

It is no wonder that since March 1, 2006, the dispensing of isotretinoin in the United States has been controlled by an FDA-mandated website called iPLEDGE—dermatologists are required to register their patients before prescribing and pharmacists are required to check the website before dispensing the drug. The prescription may not be dispensed until both parties have complied. A physician may not prescribe more than a 30-day supply, and a new prescription may not be written for at least 30 days. Pharmacies are also under similar restriction. There is also a seven-day window between the time the prescription is written and the time the medication must be picked up at the pharmacy. Doctors and pharmacists must also verify written prescriptions in an online system before patients may fill the prescription. Due to its potential to cause developmental malformations, women with the potential to bear children must commit to the use of two forms of contraception simultaneously for the duration of isotretinoin therapy, as well as for the month immediately preceding and the month immediately following therapy.[86] Alerts continue to exist against purchasing isotretinoin online.[87]

People convince themselves, and I understand their level of desperation, that these side effects are few and far between, but these side effects have affected so many people. While studies may be used to argue the likelihood of one damaging their liver or colon or the wide range of life-threatening side effects, including psychiatric problems such as depression and suicide as well as causing severe fetal deformities, miscarriages, death of the fetus and premature births, is it worth the risk?

I have a friend who was on a form of isotretinoin (generic Accutane). When I found this out, I immediately sent him a list of all the side effects, hoping that he would quit the treatment and switch to natural ways. Both he and his parents ignored the possible side effects in the same way millions of others do. Today, he has stomach and intestinal problems, including digestion problems, but excuses them as, "Oh, I just have an acid problem" or "It's just something I ate," though I wonder if the major cause was the destructive side effects of the drugs.

Some people will rave about the results they received using Accutane even though they had significant symptoms during the five- to six-month process of taking it, but the number of people who have had absolute horror stories of ruining their health makes this approach simply not worth the risk!

> *When the side effects are far worse than the results of acne, you might want to try something else.*

Don't disregard the side effect warnings. When the side effects are far worse than the results of acne, you might want to try something else. Drugs are not the only way or even the most effective way to treat acne. I encourage you to not risk a lifetime of damage to your body to heal something that will eventually go away on its own if you do nothing.

There is a far superior way.

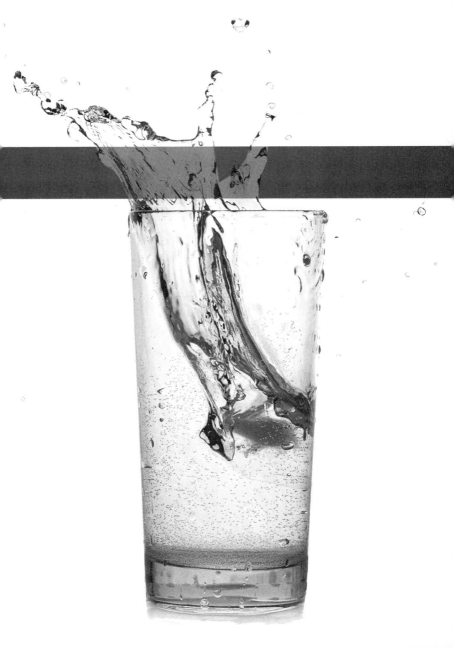

chapter 9
The Ultimate Treatment

Desperate to find a way to deal with my own acne breakouts, I went through stacks and stacks of research books and articles, making notes of my own and going through any information I could find. Through trial and error, mixing different natural ingredients together, I tried the things that seemed compelling, slowly finding what worked and what didn't work for me. I compiled my research, the summary of which you've just read through, in order to discover the system that would clear up my back and face and make my skin beautiful again.

So here is what I found that actually worked for me, and I believe will work for you.

Get Plenty of Sleep

Make sure you are getting plenty of sleep. Sleep is almost as important as breathing for your health. Sleep restores energy to the body, particularly to the brain and nervous system. The heartbeat and breathing rate slow down, blood pressure falls, muscles relax, and the overall metabolic rate of the body decreases. It is the period of the day when your hormones regulate, your body heals and recovers, having a major impact on every cell in your body. Lack of sleep adds dramatically to your stress level and will likely increase your potential for breakouts.

> *Sleep is almost as important as breathing for your health.*

Drink Plenty of Water

When you wake up in the morning, have a nice tall glass of water, preferably room temperature, and try adding a half of a lemon and a splash of apple cider vinegar, which helps to reduce or eliminate toxins in your body that may cause acne. It definitely is an acquired taste, but if you are struggling with acne, the effects are well worth putting up with the taste. As you drink, consider that more than 70 percent of your body is made up of water. Your body is constantly losing fluids that must be replenished. These fluids are crucial as to how we keep the nutrients flowing throughout our bodies and how we detoxify. You should be sipping water throughout the day with the goal of having an eight-ounce glass every waking hour or hour and a half. You should never let yourself get all the way to thirsty, because you start becoming dehydrated long before the initial thirst signal from your body. Think of dehydration as restricting the flow of fluids.

By way of contrast, it is also important to note that coffee, sodas, sweet drinks, and alcohol can actually dehydrate. Don't be fooled into thinking these liquids help keep you hydrated.

Supplement with an Antioxidant Fish Oil

Make sure you take antioxidant fish oil. This is not only crucial in your body healing the skin, but it is one of *the most important things* you can do for your health in general. The omega-3s found in fish are structural fats that make up a large portion of your brain and nervous system. Additionally, antioxidant fish oils are anti-inflammatory in nature, and quenching inflammation helps the body with flow and healing, especially the skin. I take Living Fuel's SuperEssentials Omega 3 EDA because it is the only true antioxidant fish oil of which I am aware. If you take something different, you will also need to take a full spectrum vitamin E, A, and other fat soluble antioxidants, including astaxanthin.

> *Make sure you take antioxidant fish oil.*

Dealing with an Outbreak

If you are going to pop a pimple despite dermatologists' warnings (and of course you will, who wants to leave it there?), you can actually get rid of acne faster than just leaving it alone *if you do it right.* Make sure you have done something to open your pores just prior. My personal recommendation is to go into an infrared sauna for a short time, which will get your pores wide open. Other methods are steam rooms, saunas, really hot showers or baths, and even working out. When the pores are the widest, this is when the pus will come out the smoothest and not rupture the skin as it does when you pop a zit with closed pores. *Never pop a pimple to the point of blood!* If you start to see blood, *STOP!* or it will result in scarring, and the scabs created take longer to heal than the zit itself. Be careful to not damage your skin even further than the initial problem.

Then, immediately after you pop the pimple, make sure you clean it with some form of natural antiseptic—the best being potassium iodide (SSKI) or tea tree oil, and the least effective being just soap. This will help to stop the spread of bacteria, and it will go inside and kill any bacteria still left inside the skin. If you don't pop it, rubbing in a 50-50 mixture of SSKI and DMSO (the organic sulfur compound dimethyl sulfoxide) will normally persuade the pimple or cyst to go away in a week or so. When finished with a shower, rinse with as cold of water as you can as you get out to shrink the pore sizes and not allow dirt and residues to clog them.

Don't touch, scratch, rub, itch, or wipe your face, and don't lean your head on your hands. This spreads the bacteria on the skin.

When washing and scrubbing, use something mild and organic whenever possible. The goal is not to scrape the zits off, but merely to clean the skin. Soaps with tea tree oil and aloe vera are generally perfect for the job. The gentler you can be on your skin the better, so dab to dry the skin as opposed to rubbing harshly.

After a Workout

After you work out, make sure you have something nutritious to replace all the minerals you just sweated out (I recommend Living Fuel's InSportRecovery™) as well as plenty of water to replace the loss of fluids. Finish with a shower. After this is a perfect time to gently pop any existing pimple heads, as mentioned above, and apply a germicide or antiseptic to kill any bacteria, preventing it from spreading.

Avoid Makeup

Makeup that is not organic is a chemical mess, a toxic cocktail. Not only does it clog your pores and promote further breakouts, but the chemicals throw your hormones out of whack and can cause all kinds of endocrine and other health problems. I realize it covers up existing breakouts,

> *Makeup is a chemical mess, a toxic cocktail.*

but it's best not to use any during breakouts. When you do have to wear makeup, make sure you wear organic. It may still irritate, but it doesn't have the chemical consequences of regular makeup.

Fix Your Nutrition

Fix your nutrition. Seriously, get my dad's book *The Super Health Diet*, and you'll be able to fix your nutrition for your entire lifetime. Eating dark green leafy vegetables will give you the vitamins and minerals you need, especially during periods of breakouts. Get

> *Fix your nutrition.*

your fats in line, lots of omega-3s and minimize omega-6s. NO FRIED FOODS. The best way to avoid toxin buildup in your body is to avoid eating them! Soft drinks, sweet drinks, coffee, alcohol, and smoking can contribute to toxin buildup and sludge in your body, and because they have to come out someway, your skin is a primary way.

So to avoid new breakouts, put this lifestyle in place—your sleep, hydration, and nutrition. Now it is about helping the "wounds" that you already have to heal. There are many nutrients both internal and external that can help this process.

Internal Supplements

Personally, I take the following supplements orally that are usually deficient during periods of hormonal shifts:

- Pantothenic acid
- L-Carnitine, which can reduce the amount of panathenic acid needed
- Vitamin B6
- Zinc
- Chromium
- MSM
- Curcumin
- Niacinamide

The healthier and smoother your body is operating, the quicker and more effectively it can heal.

For topical use, a mixture of aloe vera gel (with no alcohol), vitamin E oil, and vitamin A oil has been shown to be effective in helping the skin to heal. The essential oils you read about earlier are fantastic—tea tree, lavender, rose hip, bergamot. Mixing into these concoctions the vitamins I've discussed can help work wonders. You start addressing the processes that create acne internally as well as isolating the problem areas externally, and you do this naturally.

Take your health seriously. The healthier and smoother your body is operating, the quicker and more effectively it can heal.

Acne Scars

If you are like most people, once the acne is gone you will probably have some degree of scarring. The same protocols mentioned in this book are fantastic for eliminating scars over time. Scars can take longer to heal. Another huge help to speeding up the healing of scars is microneedling. This sounds painful but it really isn't. Microneedlers work by having numerous microneedles on a roller make tiny punctures in the dermis, causing blood to rush to the area with its healing factors, including stem cells, that restore the area.

Use once every week or two weeks over affected area moving the roller vertically, horizontally, and diagonally over scarred area. DO NOT USE OVER ACNE or it will just serve as a means to spread the bacteria.

After needling, use the techniques described in this book—specifically the ones topically applied to the skin—to enhance the healing process.

By now you have learned key strategies to support your body's natural processes to achieve clear youthful skin—from lifestyle modifications to the anti-inflammatory aspects of salicylic acid combined with the moisturizing and skin conditioning benefits of vitamins, minerals, essential oils, amino acids, and other natural compounds—while avoiding the use of toxic chemicals you will find in the vast majority of the products on the market today. These are the same strategies and formulations that I first used and continue to use to overcome my acne and maintain my clear skin.

For more information and to keep up with my new discoveries on acne and skin health, follow me at lxrorganics.com and LXR Organics on Facebook, Twitter, and Instagram.

Here's to clear skin and clearer skies in your future! God bless you!

Beloved, I pray that you may prosper in all things and be in health, just as your soul prospers.

The Apostle John, 3 John 2

endnotes

1 Grant RNR. "The Section of the History of Medicine: The History of Acne." *Proceedings of Royal Society of Medicine.* 1951;44;649-52.

2 Monroe H. "Acne Cures from the Past." eHow Style, Demand Media, Inc. www.ehow.com/way_5279747_acne-cures-past.htmls.

3 "History of Acne and Its Treatment." www.bestacnetreatment.org/history-of-acne-and-its-treatment.

4 Aristotle. *Historia Animalium,* 556b, 29; Problemata, 36, 3; in Ed. Casaubun (1605) pp. 654B, 639E.

5 Grant RNR. "The Section of the History of Medicine: The History of Acne." *Proceedings of Royal Society of Medicine.* 1951;44;649-52.

6 Celsius AC. *De Medicina.* Translated by Thayer; Loeb classical library edition; 1935;Vol.6;185-186.

7 Monroe H. "Acne Cures from the Past." eHow Style, Demand Media, Inc. www.ehow.com/way_5279747_acne-cures-past.htmls.

8 Haedersdal M, Togsverd-Bo K, Wulf HC. "Evidence-based review of lasers, light sources and photodynamic therapy in the treatment of acne vulgaris." *Journal of the European Academy of Dermatology and Venereology.* 2008;22(3): 267-278.

9 Doddaballapur S. "Microneedling with Dermaroller." *Journal of Cutaneous and Aesthetic Surgery.* 2009;2(2)110-11.

10 Taylor M, Gonzalez M, Porter R. (May–June 2011). "Pathways to inflammation: acne pathophysiology." *European Journal of Dermatology* 21(3):323–33. Dawson AL, Dellavalle RP. (2013). "Acne vulgaris." *BMJ* 346:f2634.

11 Arndt H, Kenneth J. (2007). *Manual of Dermatologic Therapeutics.* Lippincott Williams & Wilkins.

12 Anderson L. (2006). *Looking Good, the Australian Guide to Skin Care, Cosmetic Medicine and Cosmetic Surgery.* AMPCo. Sydney.

13 www.acne.org/adult-acne.html. Retrieved 2014-01-17.

14 www.contactmusic.com/story/adam-levine-acne-made-me-depressed_3781073. Retrieved 2014-04-15.

15 www.magweb.com/celebrity-gossip/stars-with-acne. Retrieved 2014-01-17.

16 ibid.

17 ibid.

18 ibid.

19 ibid.

20 ibid.

21 ibid.

22 http://gulfnews.com/about-gulf-news/al-nisr-portfolio/
tabloid-on-saturday/stars-acne-and-agony-1.1103474.
Retrieved 2014-01-17.

23 ibid.

24 ibid.

25 "Acne Scars." www.acne-lasertreatment.net. Retrieved
2014-01-17.

26 Watson S. "Coping with the emotional impact of acne."
www.webmd.com/skin-problems-and-treatments/acne/
acne-care-11/emotional. Retrieved 2014-01-17.

27 Goodman G. (2006). "Acne and acne scarring—the case
for active and early intervention." *Australian Family
Physician.* 35(7):503–4.

28 Magin P, Adams J, Heading G, Pond D, Smith W.
"Psychological sequelae of acne vulgaris." *Canadian Family
Physician.* 2006 August 10;52(8):979.

29 Lasek RJ, Chren M (1998). "Acne Vulgaris and the Quality
of Life of Adult Dermatology Patients." Retrieved 2014-
01-17 from http://archderm.jamanetwork.com/article.
aspx?articleid=188999.

30 ibid.

31 Hanna S, Sharma J, Klotz J. (2003). "Acne vulgaris: More than skin deep." Retrieved 2014-01-17 from http://escholarship.org/uc/item/0t2870v9.

32 Purvis D, Robinson E, Merry S, Watson P. (2006). "Acne, anxiety, depression and suicide in teenagers: A cross-sectional survey of New Zealand secondary school students." *Journal of Pediatrics and Child Health.* 42(12):793-6.

33 Tan JKL. (2008). "The Unseen Impact of Acne: There is help for those suffering." Retrieved 2014-01-17 from http://allacne.blogspot.com/2008/01/unseen-impact-of-acne-there-is-help-for.html.

34 Staff of Medindia.com. (2008, March 9). "Social Anxiety Prevents Acne Patients from Participating in Sports, Exercise." Retrieved 2014-01-17 from www.medindia.net/News/Social-Anxiety-Prevents-Acne-Patients-from-Participating-in-Sports-Exercise-33952-1.htm.

35 Krejci-Manwaring J, Kerchner K, Feldman SR, Rapp DA, Rapp SR. "Social sensitivity and acne: the role of personality in negative social consequences and quality of life." *International Journal of Psychiatry in Medicine.* 2006;36(1):121-30.

36 Tan JK, Vasey K, Fung KY. "Beliefs and Perceptions of Patients with Acne." *Journal of the American Academy of Dermatology.* 2001;44:439-45.

37 A Stanford University study showed that college students were far more likely to suffer acne flare-ups during exams than at less stressful times. Chiu A, Chon SY, Kimball, AB. "The Response of Skin Disease to Stress." *Archives of Dermatology.* 2003;139(7):897-900. doi:10.1001/arch-derm.139.7.897.

38 Craichy KC. *Super Health: 7 Golden Keys to Unlock Lifelong Vitality* (Tampa: LivingFuel Publishing, 2005), p. 55.

39 Howard D. "What Is Acne?" www.dermalinstitute.com/us/library/19_article_What_is_Acne_.html. Retrieved 2014-03-15.

40 Takayasu S, Wakimoto H, Itami S, Sano S. "Activity of testosterone 5 alpha-reductase in various tissues of human skin." *Journal of Investigative Dermatology.* 1980 Apr;74(4):187-91.

41 Howard D. "What Is Acne?" www.dermalinstitute.com/us/library/19_article_What_is_Acne_.html. Retrieved 2014-03-15.

42 Sansone G, Reisner RM. "Differential rates of conversion of testosterone to dihydrotestosterone in acne and in normal human skin—A possible pathogenic factor in acne." *Journal of Investigative Dermatology.* 1971;56:366.

43 Kaymak Y, Adisen E, Erhan M, Celik B, Gurer MA. "Zinc levels in patients with acne vulgaris." *Journal of the Turkish Academy of Dermatology.* 2007;1(3):71302a.

44 Burris J, Rietkerk W, Woolf K. "Acne: The Role of

Medical Nutrition Therapy." *Journal of the Academy of Nutrition and Dietetics.* 2013;113(3):416 DOI: 10.1016/j.jand.2012.11.016.

45 Adebamowo CA, et al. "Milk consumption and acne in adolescent girls." *Dermatology Online Journal.* 2006 May 10;12(4):1.

46 Smith RN, et al. "A low-glycemic-load diet improves symptoms in acne vulgaris patients: a randomized controlled trial." *American Journal of Clinical Nutrition.* 2007;86:107-15.

47 Quillin P, Ph.D., R.D. *Healing Nutrients* (New York: 1989, Vintage), page 377.

48 McCarthy M. "High chromium yeast for acne?" *Medical Hypotheses.* 1984:14:307-10.

49 Zouboulis CC. "Is acne vulgaris a genuine inflammatory disease?" *Dermatology.* 2001;203:277-279.

50 SJ Bhathena, E Berlin, JT Judd, YC Kim, JS Law, HN Bhagavan, R Ballard-Barbash, PP Nair. "Effects of omega 3 fatty acids and vitamin E on hormones involved in carbohydrate and lipid metabolism in men." *American Journal of Clinical Nutrition.* 1991;54:684-688.

51 Calder PC. "Dietary modification of inflammation with lipids." *Proceedings of the Nutrition Society.* 2002;61:345-358.

52 Laidlow M, Holub BJ. "Effects of supplementation with

fish oil–derived n-3 fatty acids and linolenic acid on circulating plasma lipids and fatty acid profiles in women." *American Journal of Clinical Nutrition.* Jan 2003;77:37-42.

53 Leung LH. "Pantothenic acid deficiency as the pathogenesis of acne vulgaris." *Medical Hypotheses.* 1995 Jun;44(6):490-2.

54 Leung LH. "A stone that kills two birds: How pantothenic acid unveils the mysteries of acne vulgaris and obesity." *Journal of Orthomolecular Medicine.* 1997;12(2):99-114.

55 *Springer Lexikon Kosmetik und Körperpflege.*

56 BDIH (www.kontrollierte-naturkosmetik.de/e/index_e. htm)

57 *Körterbuch der Kosmetik.*

58 El-Akawi Z, Abdel-Latif N, Abdul-Razzak K. "Does the plasma level of vitamins A and E affect acne condition?" *Clinical and Experimental Dermatology.* 2006 May;31(3):430-4.

59 *Springer Lexikon Kosmetik und Körperpflege.*

60 *Springer Lexikon Kosmetik und Körperpflege.*

61 *Körperpflegekunde und Kosmetik.*

62 http://psychcentral.com/news/archives/2006-03/msl-nss032306.html. Retrieved 2014-01-27.

63 *Springer Lexikon Kosmetik und Körperpflege.*

64 http://link.springer.com/book/10.1007/978-3-642-24688-3.

65 *Kursbuch Kosmetik.*

66 *Wörterbuch der Kosmetik.*

67 http://www.ewg.org/research/teen-girls-body-burden-hormone-altering-cosmetics-chemicals/detailed-findings. Retrieved 2014-01-21.

68 Buck Louis GM, Gray LE Jr, Marcus M, Ojeda SR, Pescovitz OH, Witchel SF, Sippell W, Abbott DH, Soto A, Tyl RW, Bourguignon JP, Skakkebaek NE, Swan SH, Golub MS, Wabitsch M, Toppari J, Euling SY. "Environmental factors and puberty timing: expert panel research needs." *Pediatrics.* 2008 Feb;121 Suppl 3:S192-207. doi: 10.1542/peds.1813E.

69 Bassett IB, Pannowitz DL, Barnetson RS. "A comparative study of tea-tree oil versus benzoyl peroxide in the treatment of acne." *The Medical Journal of Australia.* 1990 Oct 15;153(8):455-8.

70 Wallengren J. "Tea tree oil attenuates experimental contact dermatitis." *Archives of Dermatological Research.* 2011 Jul;303(5):333-8. doi: 10.1007/s00403-010-1083-y. Epub 2010 Sep 24.

71 *Körperpflegekunde und Kosmetik.*